A Guide to Mechanical Ventilation in Emergency Room

A Guide to Mechanical Ventilation in Emergency Room

2nd Edition

Kishalay Datta
MBBS MD MRCP MHA
Director and Head
Department of Emergency Medicine
Max Super Speciality Hospital
Shalimar Bagh, New Delhi, India

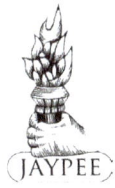

JAYPEE BROTHERS MEDICAL PUBLISHERS
The Health Sciences Publisher
New Delhi | London

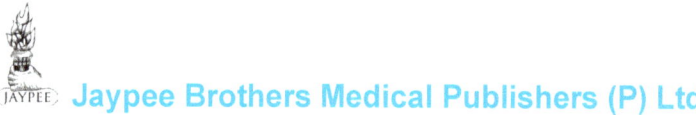
Jaypee Brothers Medical Publishers (P) Ltd

Headquarters
Jaypee Brothers Medical Publishers (P) Ltd
EMCA House, 23/23-B
Ansari Road, Daryaganj
New Delhi 110 002, India
Landline: +91-11-23272143, +91-11-23272703
+91-11-23282021, +91-11-23245672
Email: jaypee@jaypeebrothers.com

Corporate Office
Jaypee Brothers Medical Publishers (P) Ltd
4838/24, Ansari Road, Daryaganj
New Delhi 110 002, India
Phone: +91-11-43574357
Fax: +91-11-43574314
Email: jaypee@jaypeebrothers.com

Overseas Office
JP Medical Ltd
83 Victoria Street, London
SW1H 0HW (UK)
Phone: +44 20 3170 8910
Fax: +44 (0)20 3008 6180
Email: info@jpmedpub.com

Website: www.jaypeebrothers.com
Website: www.jaypeedigital.com

© 2021, Jaypee Brothers Medical Publishers

The views and opinions expressed in this book are solely those of the original contributor(s)/author(s) and do not necessarily represent those of editor(s) of the book.

All rights reserved. No part of this publication may be reproduced, stored or transmitted in any form or by any means, electronic, mechanical, photocopying, recording or otherwise, without the prior permission in writing of the publishers.

All brand names and product names used in this book are trade names, service marks, trademarks or registered trademarks of their respective owners. The publisher is not associated with any product or vendor mentioned in this book.

Medical knowledge and practice change constantly. This book is designed to provide accurate, authoritative information about the subject matter in question. However, readers are advised to check the most current information available on procedures included and check information from the manufacturer of each product to be administered, to verify the recommended dose, formula, method and duration of administration, adverse effects and contraindications. It is the responsibility of the practitioner to take all appropriate safety precautions. Neither the publisher nor the author(s)/editor(s) assume any liability for any injury and/or damage to persons or property arising from or related to use of material in this book.

This book is sold on the understanding that the publisher is not engaged in providing professional medical services. If such advice or services are required, the services of a competent medical professional should be sought.

Every effort has been made where necessary to contact holders of copyright to obtain permission to reproduce copyright material. If any have been inadvertently overlooked, the publisher will be pleased to make the necessary arrangements at the first opportunity. The **CD/DVD-ROM** (if any) provided in the sealed envelope with this book is complimentary and free of cost. **Not meant for sale.**

Inquiries for bulk sales may be solicited at: jaypee@jaypeebrothers.com

A Guide to Mechanical Ventilation in Emergency Room

First Edition: **2017**
Second Edition: **2021**
ISBN 978-93-90595-90-7

Dedicated to

My parents

Chief Contributors

Divyansh Gulati
MBBS MEM MRCEM FRCEM
Consultant
Department of Emergency Medicine
Milton Keynes Hospital
Milton Keynes, United Kingdom

Fatima Ihsan MBBS
Junior Clinical Fellow
Department of Emergency Medicine
Milton Keynes Hospital
Milton Keynes, United Kingdom

Preface to the 2nd Edition

Knowledge about principles of ventilation is a necessity, for making correct decisions in the management of acutely ill patients coming in the emergency room. The COVID-19 pandemic has taught us how ventilation can save lives.

After searching for standard literatures/research materials and books on mechanical ventilation, I felt that there was a definite need and scope for a specific book on emergency room ventilation. My efforts here are only to bring all topics related to ventilation under one roof for all medical graduates interested in mechanical ventilation.

This book will serve as a quick reference and guide for all undergraduate/postgraduate doctors/students/interns/residents/critical care nurses/technicians/respiratory physiotherapists/biomedical staffs working in the emergency room and in intensive care units.

The book deals with all necessary topics related to mechanical ventilation only. The topics are presented in a simple and easy language with all basic information, so that residents/students of Emergency Medicine can easily understand, comprehend and apply it to their patient management.

The concepts presented in this book are based on the latest available literature; but with the ever-changing facades of Emergency Medicine, these guidelines should be taken as a "guide only" to patient care.

The information presented in this book has been taken from various sources with permission. All these information along with my clinical and teaching experiences have immensely contributed to making it a better book. I would personally recommend this book to all students of mine.

Special thanks to all my teachers and students who inspired and educated me. I must thank my students and others, who were reading the texts and have contributed a lot regarding preparation of this complete new book.

I am grateful to Dr Divyansh Gulati (Oxford University Hospital Consultant) now working in Milton Keynes Hospital, Milton Keynes, United Kingdom, for immense contribution of modern literature on mechanical ventilation from different resources. He contributes one complete chapter to this book and has personally written with passion, the chapter 'Drugs used in mechanical ventilation'. The chapter is completely a new addition to this already very popular book.

Finally, I dedicate this book to my late parents Dr Jyotish Chandra Datta and Mrs Gouri Datta.

Kishalay Datta

Preface to the 1st Edition

Knowledge of principles of ventilation is a necessity, for making correct decisions in the management of acutely ill patients in the emergency room.

After searching for standard literatures and books on mechanical ventilation to teach my students, I found there was a definite need of a specific book on emergency room ventilation only. My efforts here are to bring all topics related to mechanical ventilation in the emergency room under one roof.

This book will serve as a quick reference and guide for all undergraduate students/interns/residents/doctors working in the emergency room and intensive care unit.

The book deals with all necessary topics related to ventilation only. The topics are presented in a simple and easy language with all basic information, so that residents/students of emergency medicine can easily understand, comprehend and apply it to their patient management. The concepts presented in this book are based on the latest available literature; but, with the ever-changing facades of emergency medicine, these guidelines should be taken as a "guide only" to patient care.

The information presented in this book has been taken from various sources. All these information along with my clinical and teaching experiences have immensely contributed to make it a better book. I would personally recommend to my students to read the Section 1 of the book first, followed by the Section 2. This will give them a better idea about ventilation.

Special thanks to all my students who inspire and educate me. I must thank my students Dr Indranil, Dr Rupinder, Dr Deepika, Dr Ayush, Dr Siddharth, Dr Akangsha, Dr Mohit, Dr Abid and others, who were reading the texts and have contributed a lot regarding preparation of this complete new book.

I am grateful to Dr Tamorish Kole, Professor of Emergency Medicine, Max Hospitals, New Delhi; and Dr Divyansh Gulati, Clinical Fellow, University of Oxford, UK, for helping and guiding me towards proper direction, by immensely contributing modern literature on ventilation from different sources.

Finally, I thank Rukmini Datta for immensely contributing her time and energy to this book.

Kishalay Datta

Contents

SECTION 1: BASICS OF RESPIRATION

1. **The Act of Breathing** 3
   - Control of Breathing *4*
   - Neuronal Controls of Inspiration and Expiration *8*

2. **Pulmonary Gas Exchange** 10
   - Alveolar Capillary Interface *10*
   - Gas Diffusion (As Per Fluid Dynamics Principle) *11*
   - Dead Spaces of Lungs and Ventilation/Perfusion Imbalance *13*
   - Ventilation–Perfusion Mismatch ($\dot{V}/\dot{Q}$ Mismatch) *15*

3. **Respiratory Physiology** 19
   - Lung Volumes and Capacities *19*
   - Pulmonary Dynamics *21*
   - Compliance *23*
   - Time Constants of Lungs *25*

SECTION 2: MECHANICAL VENTILATION

4. **Mechanical Ventilators** 29
5. **Initiation of Mechanical Ventilation** 31
6. **Drugs Used for Mechanical Ventilation** 33
   - Ideal Sedation Agent *33*
   - SOAPME *35*
   - Induction Agents *36*
   - Paralytic Agents *37*
7. **Ventilatory Modes** 38
   - Classification *39*
8. **Noninvasive Ventilation** 49
   - Noninvasive Ventilation or Noninvasive Positive-Pressure Ventilation *49*

9. **Inspiratory Pressures and Flow Profiles** 57
   - Inspiratory Pressures 57
   - Flow Profiles 58
10. **Pressure-Controlled Ventilation** 61
    - Pressure-Controlled Ventilation 62
11. **Positive End-Expiratory Pressure** 67
    - Auto-PEEP 68
12. **General Settings in a Ventilator** 71
    - Tidal Volume 71
    - Respiratory Rate 71
    - Minute Ventilation 72
    - Fraction of Inspired Oxygen 72
    - Positive End-Expiratory Pressure 72
    - Inspiration-Expiration Time Ratio 72
    - Flow Rate 73
    - Slope 73
    - Trigger Sensitivity 73
    - Inspiratory Peak/Plateau Pressure 74
    - Settings of Ventilator as Per Mode Selection 74
13. **Monitoring of Ventilated Patients** 76
    - Ventilator Alarms 77
14. **Ventilatory Complications in Emergency Room** 79
    - Ventilatory Complications 79
15. **Ventilator-Induced Lung Injury and Ventilator-Associated Pneumonia** 81
    - Ventilator-Induced Lung Injury 81
    - Ventilator-Associated Pneumonia 81
16. **Weaning Parameters** 86
    - Prerequisites for Weaning 87
17. **Ventilatory Strategies** 88
    - Chronic Obstructive Lung Disease/Asthma 88
    - Flail Chest 89

- Head Injury *89*
- Neuromuscular Diseases (Guillain-Barré Syndrome/ Myasthenia Gravis/Amyotrophic Lateral Sclerosis/ Myasthenia Gravis/Poliomyelitis) *90*
- Myocardial Infarction/Heart Failures/Hypovolemic Shock *90*
- Acute Respiratory Distress Syndrome *91*
- Recruitment Steps *92*

18. Ventilatory Graphics 95
- Scalar Graphics *96*
- Loop Graphics *102*

Bibliography 117

Index 133

Abbreviations

ACI	:	Alveolocapillary Interface
ACMV	:	Assist-control Mode Ventilation
BiPAP	:	Bilevel Positive Airway Pressure
$C_{Dynamic}$	:	Dynamic Compliance
CIA	:	Central Inspiratory Activity
CMV	:	Controlled Mode Ventilation
CPAP	:	Continuous Positive Airway Pressure
CSF	:	Cerebrospinal Fluid
C_{static}	:	Static Compliance
CVA	:	Cerebrovascular Accident
DRG	:	Dorsal Respiratory Group
ERV	:	Expiratory Reserve Volume
ET	:	Endotracheal Tube
FEV1	:	Forced Expiratory Volume in 1 second
FiO_2	:	Fraction of Inspired Oxygen
FVC	:	Forced Vital Capacity
[H^+]	:	Hydrogen Ion
IC	:	Inspiratory Capacity
IMV	:	Intermittent Mandatory Ventilation
IOS	:	Inspiratory Off Switch
IRV	:	Inspiratory Reserve Volume
kPa	:	Kilopascal
MV	:	Minute Ventilation
NIPPV	:	Noninvasive Positive Pressure Ventilation
NPBM	:	Nucleus Parabrachialis Medialis
PAH	:	Pulmonary Arterial Hypertension
PaO_2	:	Alveolar Partial Pressure of Oxygen
PCV	:	Pressure-controlled Ventilation
PEEP	:	Positive End-Expiratory Pressure

P_{peak}	:	Peak Inspiratory Pressure
P_{plat}	:	Plateau Inspiratory Pressure
PSV	:	Pressure Support Ventilation
R_{aw}	:	Airway Resistance
RV	:	Residual Volume
SIMV	:	Synchronized Intermittent Mandatory Ventilation
TLC	:	Total Lung Capacity
TV	:	Tidal Volume
V/Q	:	Ventilation/Perfusion
VAP	:	Ventilator-Associated Pneumonia
VC	:	Vital Capacity
VILI	:	Ventilator-Induced Lung Injury
VRG	:	Ventral Respiratory Group

SECTION

1

Basics of Respiration

1. The Act of Breathing
2. Pulmonary Gas Exchange
3. Respiratory Physiology

CHAPTER 1

The Act of Breathing

■ INTRODUCTION

The act of breathing involves an active inspiratory movement in which the chest wall is pulled outward, by contraction of intercostal muscles and downward due to descent of the diaphragm.

The control of this rhythmic respiration is under control of "centers" in brainstem, which are responsible for successive inspiration (active breathing) and expiration (passive breathing).

During inspiration, the dimensions of the thoracic cavity increase. The anteroposterior diameter (by contraction of scalene muscles), the vertical diameter (via descent of diaphragm), and the transverse diameter (via contraction of parasternal muscles) are all increased during inspiration.

This thoracic expansion in turn causes expansion of lungs, which are virtually dragged by the chest wall because of adhesive and inexpansile properties of intrapleural attachments and fluid.

This expansion of lungs naturally causes fall in "intrapulmonary pressure" within the lungs.

Once air breathed in expands the lungs, the elastic recoil of lungs also causes a slight drop in intrapleural pressure between visceral and parietal layers. This negative intrapleural pressure depends on the amount of thoracic expansion.

This intrapleural pressure (-4 to -10 cm of H_2O) varies over different regions of the lungs. The pressure is more negative at lung apices than at bases; so the negativity of intrapleural pressure will cause more expansion of lung units at apex than lower zones of lungs.

This negative intrapleural pressure results from forces within the chest wall that exerts pressure to pull the parietal pleura outward from the visceral pleura; whereas the elastic fibers of the lung exert pressure to pull visceral pleura inward from the parietal pleura.

This opposite pull of pleural layers causes pressure within the space to be subatmospheric. This negative pressure in pleural space keeps the lungs inflated.

Now due to this negative pressure formation inside the thoracic cavity as a whole, air from outside rushes into the lungs via the airways to the alveoli. The more the negative pressure, more air rushes inside the lungs. A single deep inhalation can produce negative pressures up to -18 cm of H_2O.

In expiration, relaxation of muscles (diaphragm, scalene, and intercostals mainly) occurs; the elastic coil of thoracic cavity and lungs comes back to its original state that pushes the intrapulmonary air outside the lungs.

Thus, successive cycles of inspiration and expiration continue as we breathe in and out.

■ CONTROL OF BREATHING

Control of breathing is done by a tight integrated feedback loop consisting of three components, namely:
1. Respiratory centers.
2. Respiratory sensors.
3. Respiratory effectors.

Respiratory Centers

The respiratory centers comprise of interconnected neurons situated in the medulla, pons, and lower part of the midbrain with projections to cerebral cortex (**Fig. 1**).

Respiratory centers can be classified under following heads:
- *Medullary respiratory centers*:
  - Dorsal respiratory group (DRG) neurons
  - Ventral respiratory group (VRG) neurons.
- *Pontine respiratory centers*:
  - *Apneustic centers*: These are mainly located in mid pontine regions of the brain.
  - *Pneumotaxis centers*: These are made of group of neurons (Pontine respiratory group), which inhibit actions of inspiratory centers of apneustic center. It exists mainly in lower midbrain and upper pons.

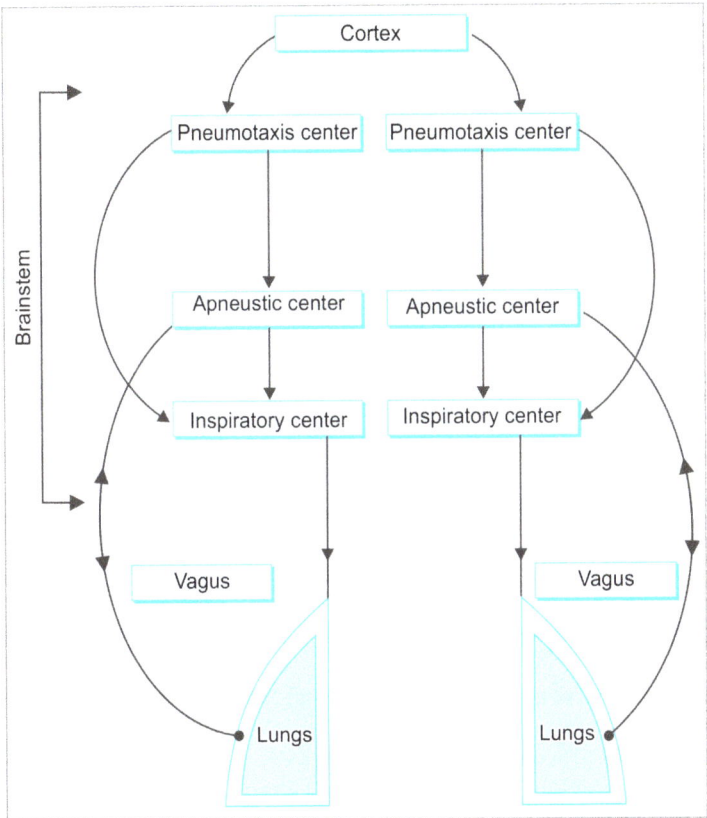

Fig. 1: Schematic diagram of respiratory centers and their connections.

- *Inspiratory and expiratory centers*: Placed more ventrally in the medulla mainly in nucleus ambiguus and nucleus retroambiguus.
- *Cerebral cortex*: The cerebral cortex functions by allowing voluntary ventilation to override the automatic controls of the medulla and pons. Voluntary ventilation control is most important during behavioral states of crying, laughing, singing, and talking. Voluntary control may override the automatic control in such states.

Both inspiratory and expiratory neurons from respiratory centers project to the intercostal and the abdominal muscles. Phrenic motor neurons and the vagus nerve supply accessory muscles of respiration **(Fig. 2)**.

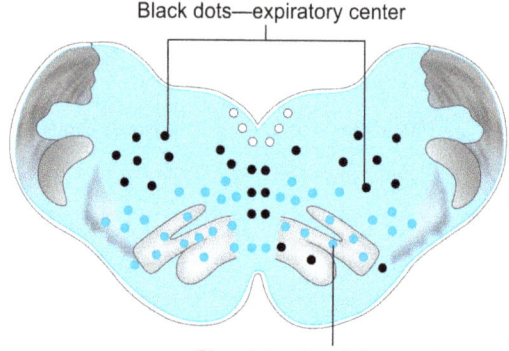

Fig. 2: Cross-section of medulla showing respiratory centers.

Thus, all these centers above serve as major control centers of respiration.

Respiratory Sensors

The respiratory sensors consist of:
- Central chemoreceptors
- Peripheral chemoreceptors
- Mechanoreceptors on chest wall and lungs.

Central Chemoreceptors

In medulla, these receptors respond rapidly to increase in [H$^+$] ion concentration in the cerebral extracellular fluid by producing linear increase in ventilation. So ventilation increases with rise in hydrogen ion concentration and vice versa.

A rise in paCO$_2$ causes movement of CO$_2$ across blood brain barrier into cerebrospinal fluid (CSF), thus stimulating the movement of hydrogen ion into extracellular fluid of brain. CO$_2$ rapidly diffuses in CSF (increasing H$^+$ ion concentration) and stimulates these chemoreceptors; so there will be rise in paCO$_2$, which will then produce immediate ventilatory response.

Compared to paCO$_2$, pH produces delayed ventilatory response due to delayed diffusion of HCO$_3$ and H$^+$ in CSF.

Peripheral Chemoreceptors

Peripheral chemoreceptors are located in aortic/carotid bodies, along the aortic arch and bifurcation of carotid arteries. They mainly respond to hypoxia (fall in levels of paO_2). Response is nonlinear. Only when paO_2 is <70 mm Hg, then respiratory stimulation occurs.

These receptors are also sensitive to variations of blood pressure. This may be the reason for increased respiratory rate in early shock where BP is low.

Mechanoreceptors

These receptors modulate forces generated during inspiration. They control rate and depth of breathing. "Tendon receptors" (in diaphragm, intercostal muscles) help in maintaining tidal volume, mainly when there is an impediment of movements of the chest wall.

Pulmonary Receptors

"Irritant receptors" (in airway epithelium): These receptors respond to chemical or physical stimuli by producing cough, bronchial constriction, and increase in ventilation.

Pulmonary stretch receptors (smooth muscles of airways): These receptors modulate to lung volumes (e.g., Hering-Breuer reflex is generally inoperative in normal conditions but gets activated when tidal volume increases twice of normal).

J receptors (in the alveolar interstitium): These respond to vascular engorgement, fluids or congestion, or fibrosis, thus producing rapid shallow breathing.

To conclude, all these receptors play an important role in controlling the rate and depth of respiration.

Respiratory Effectors

These comprise mainly of muscles of respiration **(Fig. 3)**.

Respiratory Muscles

- *Diaphragm*: Supplied by phrenic neurons ($C_{3,4,5}$) responsible for 75% of tidal volume. Most of the work of inhalation is done by this muscle.
- *External intercostal muscle, anterior serratus, sternocleidomastoid, and scalene muscles*: They play an important part in inspiratory efforts by elevating chest cage, first two ribs and sternum.
- *Abdominal muscles (oblique, rectus, and transversus)*: Exhalation is a passive process. These muscles are said to aid in expiration.

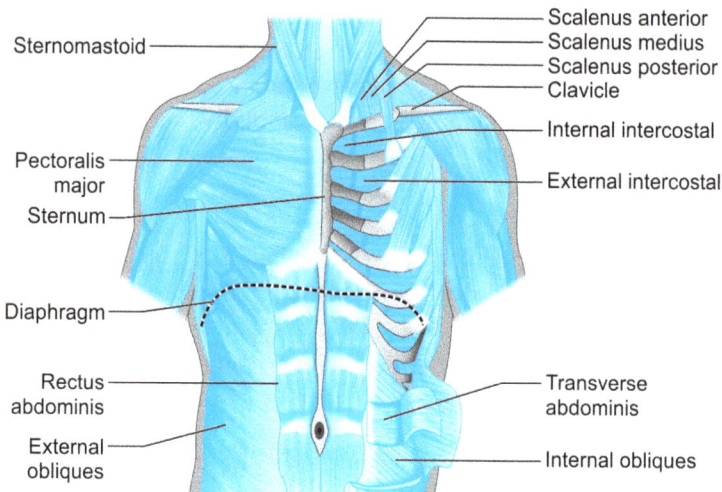

Fig. 3: Muscles of respiration.

- *Accessory muscles*: Not active during normal quiet breathing. Muscles include trapezius, pectoralis major, and scalenes.

The contractile properties of all these respiratory muscles (striated) depend on their muscle fibers and their force of contraction.

So, respiratory muscles play a pivotal role for maintenance of tidal volume and pressures, during normal process of breathing and also during diseased states which produce respiratory muscle fatigability.

NEURONAL CONTROL OF INSPIRATION AND EXPIRATION

Respiratory neurons are numerous in nucleus parabrachialis medialis (NPBM), locus coeruleus, nucleus pontis caudalis, and nucleus gigantocellularis (*all in the brainstem*). These are responsible for terminating inspiration and switching to expiration.

A slow increasing centrally generated inspiratory activity (CIA) along with discharge from pulmonary stretch receptors activates a set of "Switch Neurons" called "R_β neurons".

These switch neurons terminate inspiration and maintain inhibition of inspiratory neural discharge during subsequent expiratory phase, till expiration is completed.

Centrally generated inspiratory activity alone can attain the threshold for inspiratory off switch (IOS). IOS mechanism receives excitatory contributions from CIA, NPBM, and vagus too. Also, levels of $paCO_2$ have inhibitory effects on IOS.

To conclude, the final act of respiration (inspiration + expiration) is dependent on neuronal outputs from all three components described above via a very tight integrated feedback mechanism.

■ KEY POINTS

- A quiet inspiration may allow intrapulmonary pressures to drop by 5 mm Hg, while a deep inspiration may cause pressure drop by as much of 20 mm Hg.
- The different types of muscle fibers are:
  - *Type I*: Slow twitch fiber—highly resistant to fatigue
  - *Type IIA*: Fast twitch red fiber—very resistant to fatigue
  - *Type II B*: Fast twitch white fiber—least resistant to fatigue.
- In normal respiration, an adult breathes 6–7 L/min, breathing rate is about 8–14 breaths/min, and amount of inspired or expired air per breath is about 500 mL (approximately). Lungs have a total volume of approximately 3.5–8.5 liters.

CHAPTER 2

Pulmonary Gas Exchange

■ ALVEOLAR CAPILLARY INTERFACE

Trachea generally bifurcates into two main bronchi, which then branch to bronchioles, and then further subdivide into terminal or respiratory bronchioles **(Figs. 1A and B)**. The respiratory bronchioles give rise to alveolar ducts, which finally lead to pulmonary alveoli.

The pulmonary alveoli consist of large flat thin epithelial cells which lie in immediate proximity to numerous pulmonary capillaries forming *alveolar capillary interface (ACI)* **(Fig. 2)**.

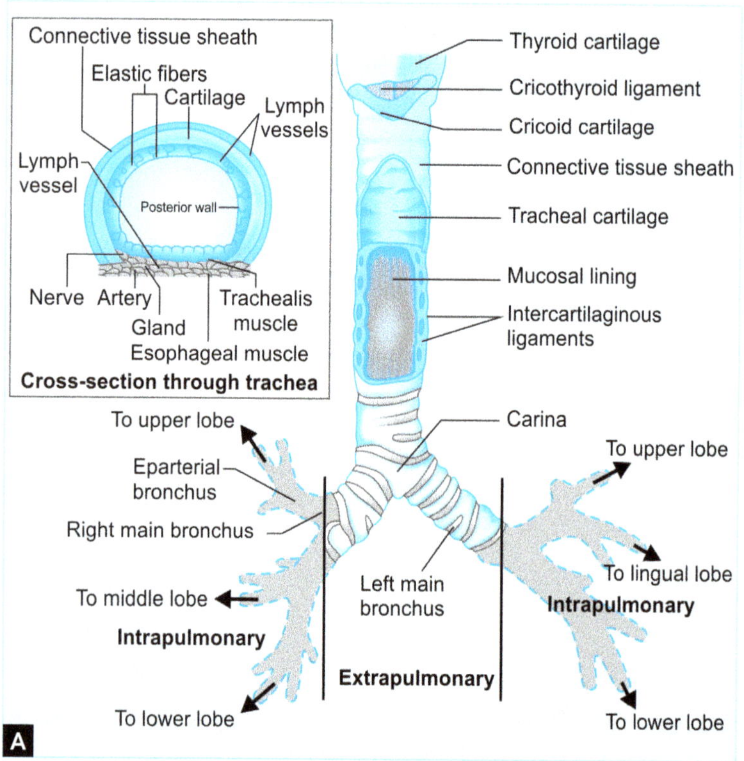

Fig. 1A

CHAPTER 2 | Pulmonary Gas Exchange

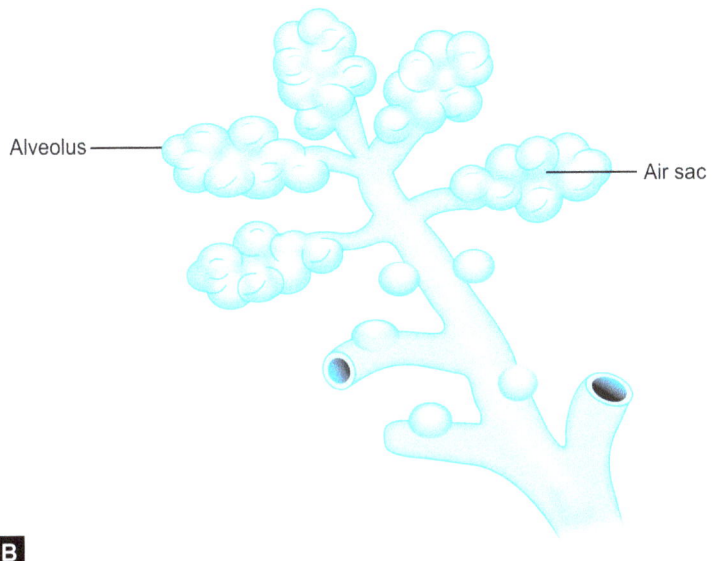

Figs. 1A and B: Respiratory bronchiole.

Pulmonary capillaries generally lie asymmetrically within walls of alveoli; so on one side, ACI is very thin allowing rapid gas exchange, while on the other side ACI is thick (interstitial space between alveolar epithelium and capillary endothelium), which allows solute and fluid exchange. Fluid from this interstitial space is drained by terminal branches of lymphatics present there.

Type II pneumocytes are located on liquid-air interface which secretes surfactant (dipalmitoylphosphatidylcholine). Surfactant acts as detergent to lower surface tension, thus reducing pressure differential to inflate the lungs and stabilize the alveoli. It acts as a water repellent layer too, preventing water penetration from capillary to alveolus.

Surfactant also contributes to anti-inflammatory and anti-microbial properties via surfactant specific proteins A, B, C, and D.

■ GAS DIFFUSION (AS PER FLUID DYNAMICS PRINCIPLE)

The rate of gas diffusion in a fluid is *directly related* to:
- Difference in the partial pressures of the gases

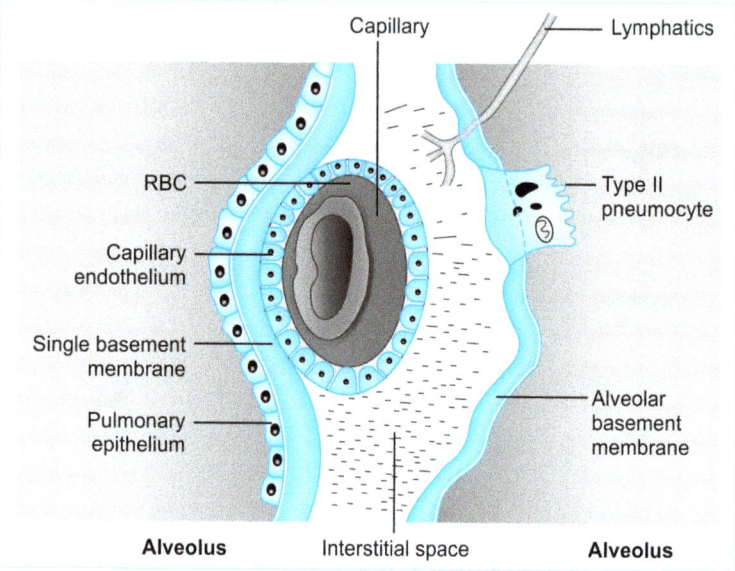

Fig. 2: Schematic view of alveolar capillary interface.

- Surface area available for diffusion of the gases
- Solubility constant (dependent on molecular weight and gas solubility of individual gases). And, *inversely related* to—distance through which the gases must diffuse.

These principles can be applied to diffusion of O_2 and CO_2 through ACI.

Difference in Partial Pressures of Gases (O_2 and CO_2) in Lungs (Fig. 3)

Gases diffuse from higher to lower pressures.

Surface Area of Lungs

The total diffusion surface area of lung is enormous (160 m^2) and very thin (0.3–0.7 micrometers). Diseases like pneumonia, emphysema, and atelectasis reduce this surface area.

Solubility Constant Depending on Gas Solubility

O_2, CO_2, and nitrogen are highly lipid soluble, so they are easily soluble in cell membranes which consist of lipids.

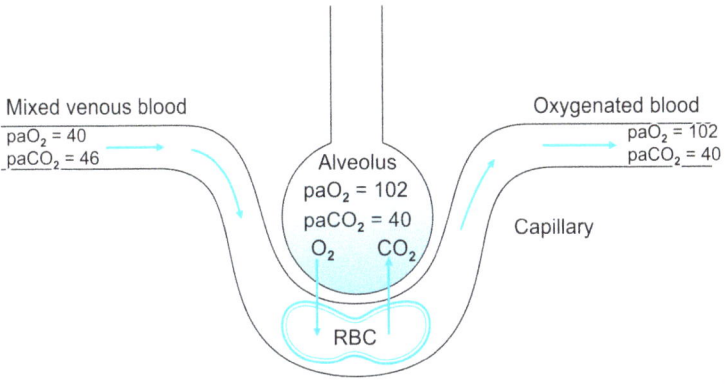

Fig. 3: Gas exchange in alveolar capillary interface.
(RBC: red blood cell)

O_2 and CO_2 are exchanged from higher gas pressure to relatively lower gas pressures by diffusion across ACI.

CO_2 is more soluble than O_2 and O_2 is twice more soluble than N_2 (nitrogen) in lipids.

Diffusion Distance in Lungs

Diffusion surface thickness of lungs varies between 0.3 and 0.7 mm. So gases diffuse very fast. The diameter of pulmonary capillaries is less than 0.8 mm. Red blood cells (RBCs) has to squeeze through these capillaries.

As RBCs surface comes in contact with the capillary surface, O_2 directly passes into RBC without going through the plasma. This brings down diffusion distance (e.g., pulmonary edema increases diffusion distance resulting in poor gaseous exchange) **(Fig. 4)**.

DEAD SPACES OF LUNGS AND VENTILATION/ PERFUSION IMBALANCE

- *Dead space of lungs can be categorized as*:
    - Anatomical dead space
    - Physiological dead space.

Anatomical dead space: It includes all airways (upper airways, bronchi, and bronchioles) that do not take part in gaseous exchange.

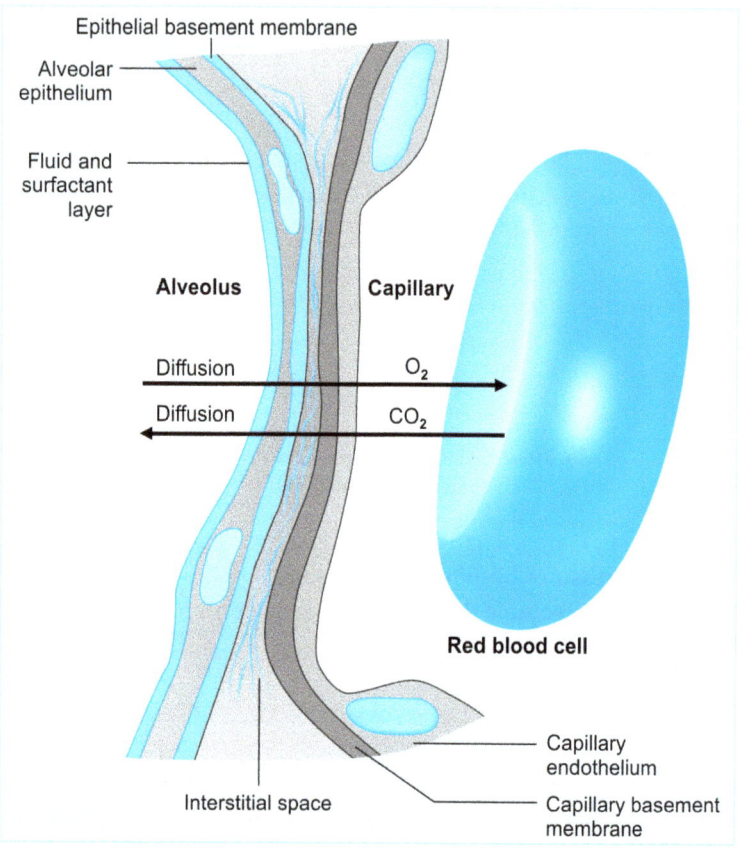

Fig. 4: Diffusion distance in lungs.

Physiological dead space: It includes all anatomical dead space plus alveolar spaces that receive air, but because of perfusion, irregularities do not participate in gaseous exchange:

- *Alveolar-arterial oxygen gradient:* It calculates the difference between alveolar PO_2 (PAO_2) and arterial PO_2 (paO_2), which occurs due to "diffusion defects" or "V-Q imbalance". It gives a good estimate of impairment of alveolar function.

It is calculated in clinical practice as $P(A-a)\ O_2 = 147 - (paCO_2 \times 1.25) - paCO_2$.

- *Diffusion defects:* These cause problems in diffusion across ACI. O_2 and CO_2 move across ACI from higher pressure to lower pressure very fast. So, diseases manifested by diffusion barrier or block (pulmonary fibrosis, pulmonary edema) may cause significant CO_2 retention and hypoxemia.

■ VENTILATION–PERFUSION MISMATCH ($\dot{V}/\dot{Q}$ MISMATCH)

The term ($\dot{V}/\dot{Q}$) or ventilation—perfusion refers to the amount of air entering alveoli per minute relative to capillary perfusion of those alveoli in a minute.

A $\dot{V}/\dot{Q}$ ratio of 1.0 means the amount of ventilation in an alveolar unit (e.g., 1 mL/min) is available for exchange of gases with equal amount of capillary blood in that unit (1 mL/min) **(Fig. 5)**. Normally, alveolar ventilation is approximately 4 L/min. and pulmonary capillary perfusion is approximately 5 L/min. So the normal ventilation/perfusion ratio is 4:5 or 0.8.

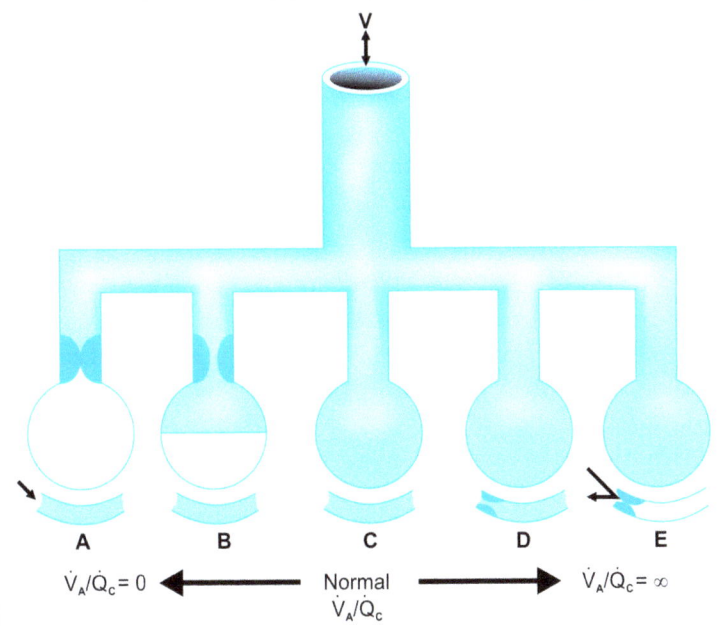

Fig. 5: Continuum of ventilation/perfusion ($\dot{V}/\dot{Q}$) relationships. (A) Intrapulmonary shunting; (B) $\dot{V}/\dot{Q}$ mismatching is a shunt-producing situation; (C) Normal $\dot{V}/\dot{Q}$ ratio; (D) $\dot{V}/\dot{Q}$ mismatching is a dead space-producing situation; and (E) Alveolar dead space.
Source: Misasi RS, Keyes JL. Matching and mismatching ventilation and perfusion in the lung. Crit Care Nurse. 1996;16(3):23.

Various factors can play a role affecting the matching between ventilation and perfusion, and their relationship should be taken as continuum. At one end of continuum, alveolus is receiving ventilation but not receiving any perfusion; resulting in its inability to participate in gaseous exchange, thus producing *alveolar dead space*. On the other end of the continuum, alveolus is receiving perfusion, but no ventilation resulting in no participation of gaseous exchange. This situation is known as *intrapulmonary shunting*.

An infinite number of ventilation/perfusion mismatches exist between the above extremes of the continuum. Situations where ventilation exceeds perfusion ($\dot{V}/\dot{Q} > 0.8$) are considered to be *dead space producing*. Whereas, situations in which perfusion exceeds ventilation ($\dot{V}/\dot{Q} < 0.8$) are considered to be *shunt producing*.

From the schematic diagram below, we can consider $\dot{V}/\dot{Q}$ functions under these four categories:

1. Normal $\dot{V}/\dot{Q}$ (intact ventilation, intact perfusion) therefore $\dot{V}/\dot{Q} = 1/1 = 1$.
2. *Ventilation without perfusion*: $V/0 = \infty$ infinity (e.g., dead space ventilation).
3. *Perfusion without ventilation*: $0/P = 0$ (e.g., shunt).
4. No perfusion, no ventilation.

Low $\dot{V}/\dot{Q}$ mismatch: This is said to exist if ventilation is reduced in proportion to perfusion. This is the most common type of $\dot{V}/\dot{Q}$ mismatch. Some group of alveoli may be poorly ventilated, while some other groups may be properly ventilated in a diseased state.

Ultimately what matters is uniformity of ventilation and perfusion.

Hypoxia can be corrected in low $\dot{V}/\dot{Q}$ mismatch by supplemental O_2 (e.g., pneumonia).

High $\dot{V}/\dot{Q}$ mismatch: This is said to exist if perfusion is reduced in proportion to ventilation. Here $\dot{V}/\dot{Q}$ ratio is zero and supplemental O_2 will not raise arterial O_2 tension (correction of hypoxia), since O_2 is not able to access blood because of no perfusion **(Fig. 6)**.

When $\dot{V}/\dot{Q}$ is zero, it is called colloquially a "*SHUNT*"—though the correct terminology is "right-to-left shunt of pulmonary capillary blood". A shunt is therefore an extreme $\dot{V}/\dot{Q}$ imbalance (e.g., in pulmonary embolism).

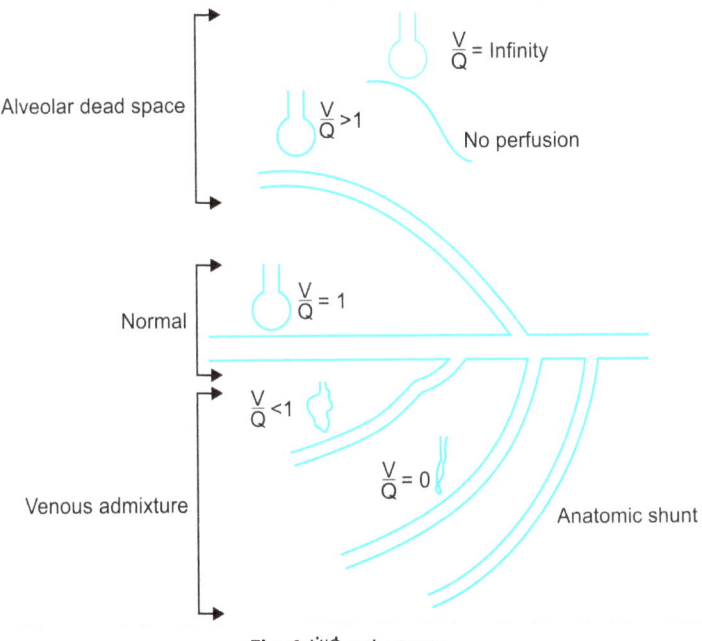

Fig. 6: V̇/Q̇ ratio range.

It is paramount to know that pulmonary vasculature has ability to alter its circulation by limiting blood flow to areas of low O_2 concentration and thus reducing right to left shunt via vasoconstriction.

The distribution of ventilation throughout lungs is uneven due to several factors like gravity and sizes of thoracic cavity. The thoracic cavity allows more lung expansion at bases than apices. Gravity also makes regional variations of intrapleural pressures. Alveoli at apices are generally larger than bases and have more air left in them during expiration compared to base. So, alveoli at apex is more difficult to inflate and less compliant normally. In upright position, alveoli at bases receive four times more ventilation than apex. In supine position, similar effects also occur on posterior dependent zones.

Perfusion distributions are also related to gravity and intra-alveolar pressures. Due to gravity, perfusion pressures in bases of lung are higher than apices. So, preferential high blood flow is seen at bases compared to apices. In some areas of lungs, intra-alveolar

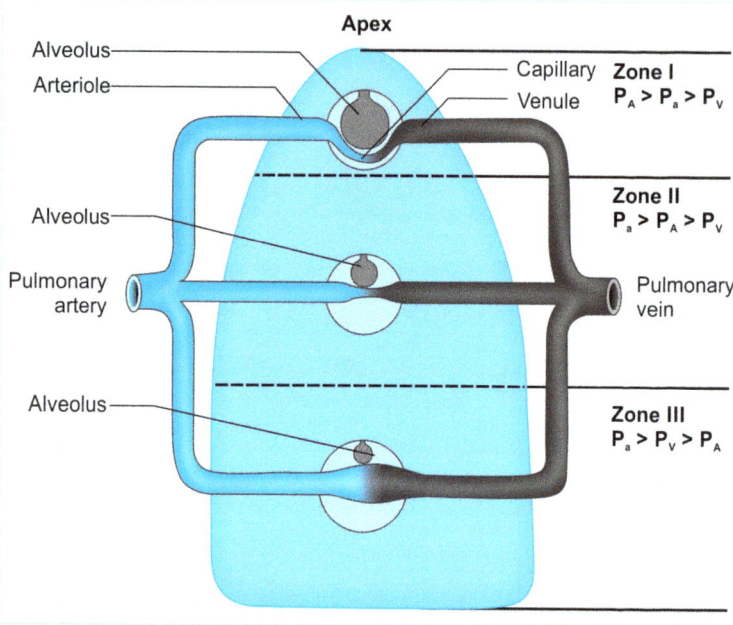

Fig. 7: Different perfusion zones of lung.

pressures have the potential to exceed capillary hydrostatic pressure. Based on this concept, lungs can be divided in three zones **(Fig. 7)**:

- *Zone 1*: It is the nondependent portion of lung which has potential for no perfusion.
- *Zone 2*: It is the middle portion of lung which receives various degrees of blood flow.
- *Zone 3*: It is the gravity dependent part of lung which receives a constant blood flow.

■ KEY POINTS

- *Normal values*:
  (1 kilo pascal = 7.5 mm Hg)
  paO_2 10.5–13.5 kPa
  $paCO_2$ 4.5–6 kPa
  pH   7.35 to 7.45
- *Severe hypoxia*:   <8 kPa
- *Type I respiratory failure*: paO_2 < 8 kPa and $paCO_2$ < 6.0 kPa
- *Type II respiratory failure*: $paCO_2$ > 6.0 kPa and paO_2 < 8 kPa
- Normal level is <15 mm Hg at 20 years, and increases by 4 mm Hg every decade.

CHAPTER 3: Respiratory Physiology

LUNG VOLUMES AND CAPACITIES

Lung volumes can be classified into static and dynamic volumes:
- *Static volumes* **(Fig. 1)**: These are as follows:
  - *Total lung capacity (TLC)*: It is the total volume of air in lungs at full inspiration.
  - *Vital capacity (VC)*: This is the volume of air expired from full inspiration to full expiration (3–6 L approx).
  - *Residual volume (RV)*: This is the volume left in the lung even after breathing out VC.
  - *Tidal volume (TV)*: It is the volume inspired or expired with each breath at rest.

Total lung capacity **(Fig. 2)**:
TLC = IRV + TV + ERV + RV
    = VC + RV

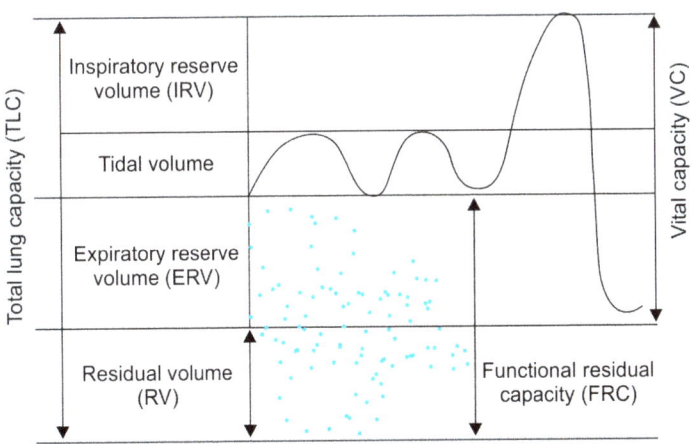

Fig. 1: Static volumes of respiratory system.

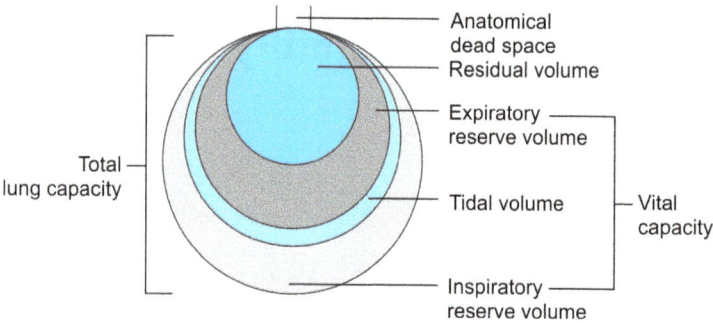

Fig. 2: Total lung volume.

TLC is normally,

    Male 6,000 mL (approximately);
    Female 4,000 mL (approximately)
    IRV = 3,000 mL (approximately)

Functional residual capacity:
FRC = ERV + RV

    ERV = 1,000 mL (approximately)
    RV = 1,500 mL (approximately);
    FRC = 2,500 mL (approximately)

Inspiratory capacity:
IC = IRV + TV

    VC is normally in
    Male 4,500 mL (approximately);
    Female 3,500 mL (approximately)

Vital capacity:
VC = IRV + TV + ERV
    = IC + ERV

- *Dynamic volumes*: These are measured because these volumes change with breathing.
  Spirometry measures functional lung volumes of lungs.
- *Forced vital capacity (FVC)*: This is the forced maximal volume of air expired from full inspiration (TLC) to full expiration (RV), when the patients is breathing out as hard and long as he can.
- *Forced expiratory volume over 1 second (FEV1)*: This is the amount of the air expired over first second of FVC. Normally, FEV1 is >75–80% of (VC). The normal FEV1/FVC ratio is normally around 70–80%. This is measured by spirometry and helps to differentiate between obstructive and restrictive lung diseases.

Figure 3 shows volume of air breathed out in first second of forced expiration (FEV1) which is over 70% of FVC.

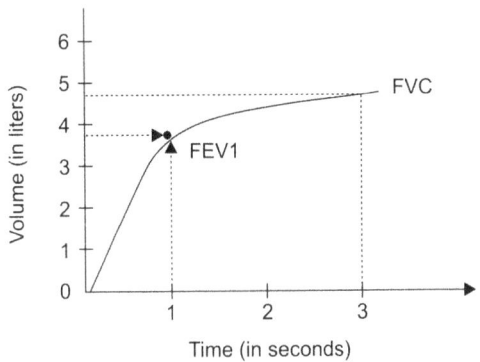

Fig. 3: Volume of air breathed out in first second of forced expiration. (FEV1: forced expiratory volume over 1 second; FVC: forced vital capacity)

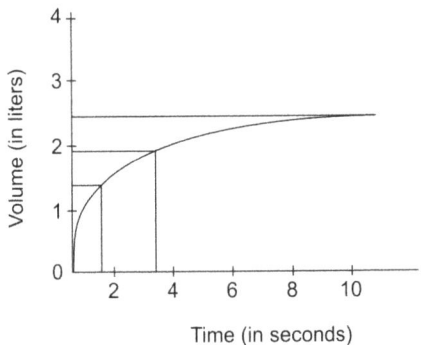

Fig. 4: In obstructive lung disease, FEV1/FVC ratio is reduced. (FEV1: forced expiratory volume over 1 second; FVC: forced vital capacity)

In *obstructive lung diseases*, time taken to fully expire is prolonged, and FEV1/FVC ratio is reduced **(Fig. 4)**.

Long time (>10 seconds) is needed to expire and both FEV1/FVC are reduced.

In *restrictive diseases of lungs*, both FEV1 and FVC are reduced proportionally but ratio of FEV1/FVC remains same even though absolute values are reduced **(Fig. 5)**.

■ PULMONARY DYNAMICS

Airway resistance (R_{aw}) is defined by the ratio of driving pressure of gas against flow.

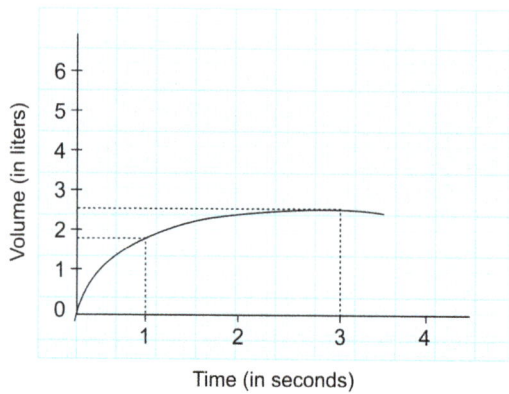

Fig. 5: In restrictive disease of lungs, both FEV1 (forced expiratory volume over 1 second) and FVC (forced vital capacity) are reduced proportionately.

In relation to airways,

$$R_{aw} = \Delta P/V$$

where ΔP = Pressure difference across an airway and V = Airflow. As per fluid dynamics notation:

"Poiseuille's Law" states $\Delta P = 8\ \mu LQ/\pi r^4$

where ΔP = Pressure loss, L = Length of pipe, μ = Dynamic viscosity, Q = Volumetric flow rate, r = Radius of pipe, π = Mathematical constant Pi.

This "Poiseuille's Law" has been applied to respiratory tract physiology, to calculate the resistance of fluids (gases) flowing through long and narrow tubes (airways).

So as per the law, airway resistance is calculated as:

$$R_{aw} = 8\ \mu L/\pi r^4$$

where μ = Viscosity of gases, L = Length of tube, r = Radius of tube, π = Mathematical constant.

If the viscosity of fluid (O_2 and air mixture viscosity is constant in a ventilator circuit) and length of tube [endotracheal (ET) is 25–26 cm long] is constant, then the flow is inversely proportional to the radius to power four. Thus, if airway radius is reduced by 50%, the resistance is increased and flow is reduced by 16-fold.

The autonomic nervous system innervates the smooth muscles found in the wall of airways from trachea to terminal bronchioles. A combination of both parasympathetic and sympathetic innervations acts to maintain the airway diameter by constriction of vessels by smooth muscles and increased mucus production.

Thus, "radius" is a powerful determinant of airway resistance. A decrease in radius will vastly increase airway resistance leading to detrimental lung mechanics.

Now consider an ET tube, which is neither long nor straight; we can assume that ET will not be suitable for smooth (laminar) flow of air inside it. Further, bend of ET will not contribute to laminar flow instead will produce turbulence.

The secretions and encrustations inside ET will also decrease the diameter in a sick patient. All these together will contribute to an increased resistance. Ultimately, increased airway resistance to airflow will lead to increased work of breathing.

To conclude the role of ET in airway, resistance should always be kept in mind during ventilation.

In a ventilator airway, resistance can be calculated as:

$$R_{aw} = (P_{peak} - P_{plat})/V$$

P_{peak} --------------- > Peak airway pressure
P_{plat} --------------- > Plateau inspiratory pressure
V --------------> Flow (volume per unit time)

For example, if peak pressure is 20 cm H_2O and plateau pressure is 18 cm H_2O and V = 60 L/min (since 1 L/1 second), therefore,
$R_{aw} = (20-18)/1 = 2$ cm $H_2O/L/s$.

■ COMPLIANCE

Compliance describes the relationship between lung volume (V) and pressure (P).

It is the change in volume (ΔV) per unit change in pressure (ΔP). So, compliance = $\Delta P/\Delta V$.

Compliance of lung is measured as how easily a lung can be distended with air pressure. So, if the lungs can be easily distended with a small amount of airway pressure—they are said to be *"Highly compliant."*

Now a graphical representation of compliance of lungs can be derived from pressure-volume curve **(Fig. 6)**.

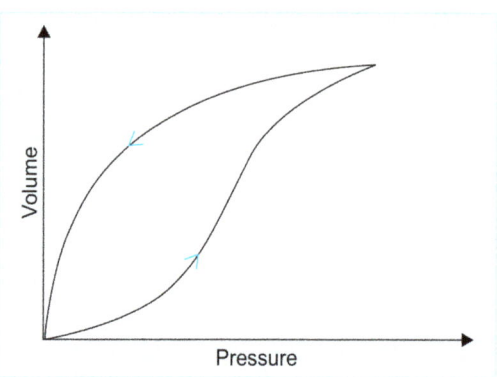

Fig. 6: Normal pressure—volume curve.

The pressure–volume curve which is obtained by plotting changes of pressure in X-axis and volume in Y-axis is relatively flat and horizontal in upper and lower portions.

In normal healthy condition of lungs, the lung operates on middle steep part of pressure—volume curve.

At very low and high volumes, the lung has to operate on lower and upper flat portions of curve respectively, where significant pressure is needed for a significant change in volume. So, the work of breathing increases in lower and upper portions of the curve thus making the lungs less compliant.

Compliance can be divided further into:
- Static compliance
- Dynamic compliance.

Static Compliance

This is the change in lung volume per unit change in pressure across the lung. In other words, it measures distensibility of respiratory system (lung plus chest wall). In ventilated patients, the static compliance of a patient with normal lungs and chest wall varies between 60 and 100 mL/cm H_2O. Decrease of static compliance below 30 mL/cm H_2O increases work of breathing.

Static compliance can be measured in a ventilator by the formula (*see* Chapter 8).

where,

$$C_{static} = V/P_{plat} - PEEP$$

V = Tidal volume, P_{plat} = Plateau pressure

Static compliance is decreased in interstitial lung diseases, pulmonary edema, pneumonia, etc.

Dynamic Compliance

It reflects lung and chest wall stiffness, along with airway resistance, when breathing occurs.

So, it is a measure of both "static compliance" and "airway resistance".

Therefore, dynamic compliance decreases when lung stiffness increases and also when airway resistance increases.

Dynamic compliance in a ventilator can be calculated as (*see* Chapter 8).

where,
$$C_{Dynamic} = V/P_{Peak} - PEEP$$

V = Tidal volume, P_{Peak} = Peak inflation pressure

Dynamic compliance can decrease due to airway obstruction.

Causes

- Blocking of ET by secretions and clot
- Heat moisture exchange filters getting blocked
- Bronchospasm
- Biting of ET (tube) by patient.

Both static and dynamic compliance can be assessed from ventilator graphics, which are demonstrated in a graphical form in **Figure 7**.

■ TIME CONSTANTS OF LUNGS

The rate at which an individual lung unit fills is known as "time constant". Five "time constants" are needed for a lung to completely fill or empty.

So, 1st time 1st constant (time offered) fills or empties 65% of lungs, 2nd time 2nd constant (time offered) fills or empties 85% of lungs, 3rd time 3rd constant (time offered) fills or empties 95% of lungs, 4th time 4th constant (time offered) fills or empties 98% of lungs, and 5th time 5th constant (time offered) fills or empties 100% of lungs.

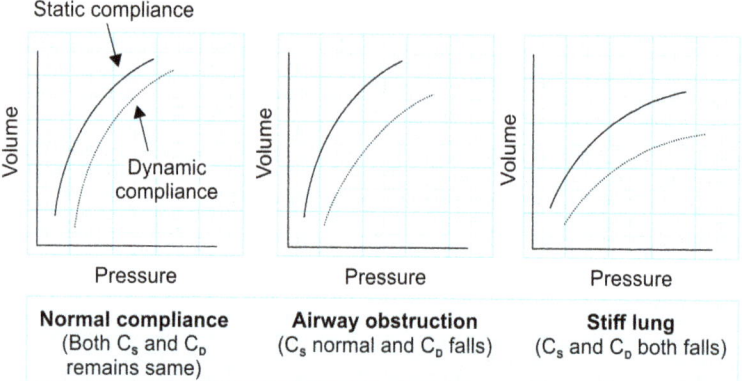

Fig. 7: Normal compliance airway obstruction stiff lung.

So, five times (compliance × resistance) gives the time for 100% filling/emptying of the lung units, respectively.

Now suppose in a ventilator, airway resistance is 1 cm $H_2O/L/s$ and compliance 0.1 $L/cm/H_2O$. So time constant is $1 \times 0.1 = 0.1$ second. So,

0.1 s × 5 = 0.5 seconds are needed to fill or empty lung units. While setting.

I:E ratio of the ventilator, this time constant is necessary to remember.

■ KEY POINTS

- There are lots of limitations and differences when "Poiseuille's Law" is applied to human respiratory tract.
- About 90–95% airway resistance originates in airways having >2.0 mm diameter.
- Normal R_{aw} ranges from 0.5–2.5 cm $H_2O/L/s$.
- ET increases R_{aw} to 6 cm $H_2O/L/s$. In COPD/asthma airway resistance may vary from 5 to 20 cm $H_2O/L/s$.
- Tracheostomy tube, with shorter length with an identical diameter of ET, does not contribute much to decrease in airway resistance.

SECTION 2

Mechanical Ventilation

4. Mechanical Ventilators
5. Initiation of Mechanical Ventilation
6. Drugs Used for Mechanical Ventilation
7. Ventilatory Modes
8. Noninvasive Ventilation
9. Inspiratory Pressures and Flow Profiles
10. Pressure-Controlled Ventilation
11. Positive End-Expiratory Pressure
12. General Settings in a Ventilator
13. Monitoring of Ventilated Patients
14. Ventilatory Complications in Emergency Room
15. Ventilator-Induced Lung Injury and Ventilator-Associated Pneumonia
16. Weaning Parameters
17. Ventilatory Strategies
18. Ventilatory Graphics

CHAPTER 4

Mechanical Ventilators

■ INTRODUCTION

Mechanical ventilators are devices, which deliver gases (air and oxygen mixture generally) to patient's airways in a controlled manner.

These devices generate a "positive pressure" at airway opening and push air into the patient's lungs. During positive pressure ventilation, airway pressure is raised above the atmospheric pressure, thus forcing air into the respiratory tract. Expiration is always passive.

Positive pressure ventilation can be applied in an "invasive manner" (via a tube in patient's airway) or "noninvasive manner" via an interface (nasal masks/orofacial masks/helmets).

Modern ventilators have the ability to monitor patient's all necessary ventilatory requirements. Delivered breath parameters, patient's response, device malfunction, and other parameters, can all be monitored with the help of active sensors, sophisticated alarms, and feedback systems in the ventilator.

All parameters of ventilatory requirements can be set on the ventilators control panel. The O_2 and compressed air from wall outlets are mixed; then this air and O_2 mixture enters patient's airways through the inspiratory tubes of the ventilator.

The exhaled air comes back to ventilator via expiratory tubes (polyvinyl corrugated tubes) and is discharged outside into the atmosphere through the expiratory port of the ventilator.

Generally, a ventilatory circuit consists of the following components **(Fig. 1)**:

- *Viral/bacterial filters*: These are mechanical filters with hydrophobic membrane of coated glass fibers. Due to hydrophobicity, potential contaminated fluids such as blood, condensate, sputum, and bacteria cannot pass to the patient's airway. Further, they inhibit airborne/fluid-borne passage of microorganisms.

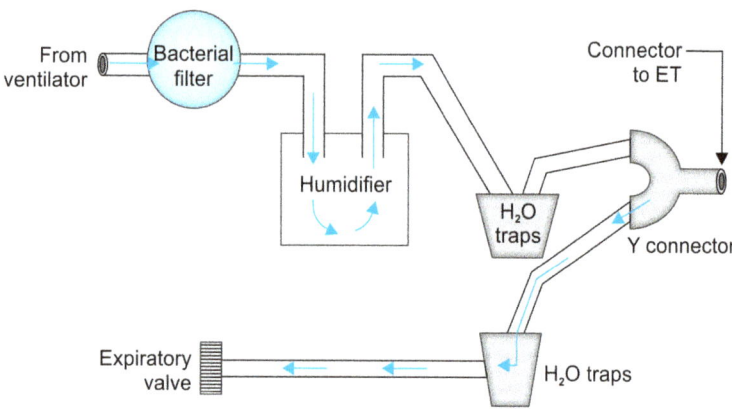

Fig. 1: A schematic representation of a ventilator circuit. (ET: endotracheal)

These filters are also common site for air-leakage in ventilator circuit. Newer technologies are nowadays increasingly being used to make these filters.

- *Humidifiers*: These are the devices that generate water vapor or steam to increase the moisture levels in the air (humidity). Thus, they prevent dryness of airways resulting in less irritation of airways.

This is the most common site for air leakage in a ventilatory circuit.

- *Water traps*: Generally one or two water traps are used in the circuit. They trap excess water in the circuit. Air leakage is very common from these sites.
- *The "Y connector"*: It has a port for temperature monitoring. The other end of this "connector" has a universal connector that connects to all endotracheal/tracheostomy tubes and other interfaces.
- *Expiratory valve*: Closure of internally situated exhalation valve (inside the ventilator) directs the air and oxygen mixture to the patient in a controlled manner via the inspiratory circuit. This valve opens after each inspiration, thus permitting exhalation. Misalignment of expiratory flap valve is a gross leak point, which may throw the ventilator out of service.
- *Interconnecting polyvinyl-corrugated tubes*: These connect the ventilator to patient's tube (endotracheal/tracheostomy) and constitute both inspiratory and expiratory limbs of the ventilator.

CHAPTER 5
Initiation of Mechanical Ventilation

INTRODUCTION

Mechanical ventilatory support is generally indicated in critically ill patients, whose respiratory effort is not sufficient to maintain their life.

Classically, indications for initiation of mechanical ventilation in such patients can be subdivided under three major heads:
1. *Hypoxia*: It is insufficient delivery of oxygen to tissues. It is arbitrarily defined as $paO_2 < 60$ mm of Hg.
2. *High work of breathing (WOB)*: Increased work of respiratory muscles can increase WOB, which may result in hemodynamic compromise of the patient.
3. *Hypoventilation*: A rising $paCO_2$ occurs due to hypoventilation.

Also, mechanical ventilation after intubation can be initiated under the following situations:
- Airway protection or securing the airway in a sick patient
- Depressed sensorium (Glasgow Coma Score < 8)
- Sudden hemodynamic compromise occurring in a patient
- Sudden cardiorespiratory arrest
- Injury to airways, chest, and facial region causing difficulty in breathing
- *Special situations*:
  - Heavy sedation for procedures
  - Transportation
- *Respiratory muscle dysfunction*:
  - Respiratory muscle fatigue
  - Neuromuscular disease
  - Increased airway resistance
- Failure of noninvasive ventilation (NIV) in patients.

Based on *pulmonary mechanics criteria*, mechanical ventilation can also be initiated when:
- FEV1 < 10 mL/kg body weight
- FVC < 15 mL/kg body weight (can be assessed by spirometer)

- Respiratory rate > 35 breaths/min
- $paCO_2$ > 60 mm Hg (if rising and in presence of acidemia)
- paO_2 < 60 mm Hg [on 40% O_2 and widened (A-a) O_2 gradient].

It must always be remembered that all these indications/criteria mentioned for initiation of ventilation above, serve as a guide only.

The treating doctor/caregiver has to take all clinical situations under consideration, before going ahead with intubation and initiation of mechanical ventilation.

Alternatively, the patient may not satisfy every criterion for invasive ventilatory management and yet has to be intubated and ventilated.

Considering all of the above-mentioned parameters, it should be kept in mind, as an emergency physician, the primary indication is to intubate early, when the doctor at the best of his judgment thinks, it is necessary to intubate and ventilate the patient.

Drugs Used for Mechanical Ventilation

CHAPTER 6

▪ IDEAL SEDATION AGENT

The ideal sedation agent does not exist as mechanical ventilation is a dynamic process and therefore largely depends on the physiological variants of the patient. Features of the hypothetical ideal sedation agent are:

- *Pharmaceutics*:
  - Ease of administration
  - Does not promote growth of pathogens
  - Easily prepared and long shelf life.
- *Pharmacodynamics*:
  - Predictable dose-dependent effects with minimal individual variation
  - Provides appropriate sedation, anxiolysis, amnesia, and analgesia
  - No tolerance and withdrawal symptoms
  - Provides facilitation of ventilator synchrony and the performance of various procedures and nursing interventions.
- *Pharmacokinetics*:
  - Rapid onset of action
  - Easily titratable level of adequate sedation
  - Short-acting, allowing patient assessment, rapid recovery following discontinuation, easy weaning from mechanical ventilation, and early extubation
  - Minimal metabolism; not dependent on normal hepatic, renal, or pulmonary function
  - No active or toxic metabolites
  - Safe for all ages with no age-related changes in pharmacokinetics
  - Lack of accumulation with prolonged administration.
- *Interactions*: No or minimal interactions with other drugs.

Flowchart 1: Types of general anesthetics.

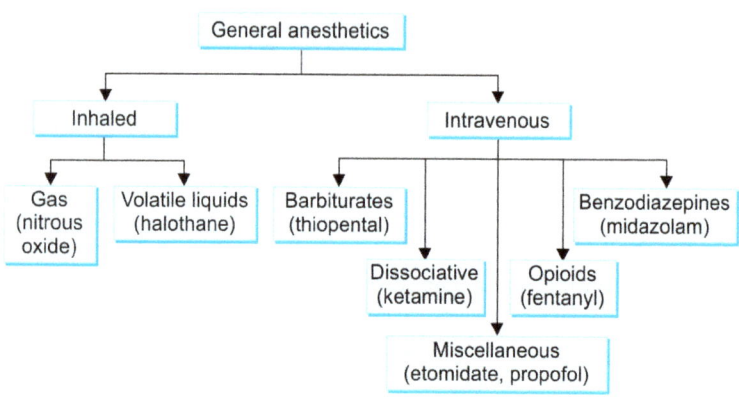

- *No or few adverse effects*:
  - No anaphylaxis or allergic reaction
  - No nausea, vomiting, or phlebitis
  - Minimal respiratory depression
  - Minimal effect on cardiovascular function
  - No pain on injection
  - No suppression of cortisol production by the adrenal cortex.
- *Other*:
  - Cost-effective
  - Lack of abuse potential
  - Widely available.[1]

General anesthetics can be divided as shown in **Flowchart 1**.[2]

Mode of Administration

Drugs given to induce general anesthesia can be either as gases or vapors (inhalational anesthetics), or as injections [intravenous (IV) anesthetics or even intramuscular (IM)]. All of these agents share the property of being quite hydrophobic (i.e., as liquids, they are not freely miscible—or mixable—in water, and as gases they dissolve in oils better than in water). It is possible to deliver anesthesia solely by inhalation or injection, but most commonly the two forms are combined, with an injection given to induce anesthesia and a gas used to maintain it.

Drugs Used during Mechanical Ventilation

In general, patients who are receiving mechanical ventilation via endotracheal (ET) tube may require the following medications:
- Sedatives
- Analgesics
- Paralytics

Examples of Drugs Used in Mechanical Ventilation

Here are some examples of sedative, analgesic, and paralytic medications that are used during mechanical ventilation (**Table 1**).[3]

Rapid Sequence Intubation

In an emergency department (ED), since controlling the airway is the priority and time is an extremely important factor therefore we mainly use IV anesthetic agents.

Before administrating the drugs for rapid sequence intubation (RSI), remember preparation is a significant step.

■ SOAPME

S—Suction
O—*Oxygen*: Bag valve mask and nonrebreathing mask with high flow oxygen
A—*Airways*: Appropriate size ET tube with bougie, laryngoscopes, and subsequent plans if anticipating difficult airway (surgical airway set)
P—Preoxygenation

TABLE 1: Drugs for mechanical ventilation.

Drug type	Examples
Sedatives	Propofol Lorazepam Midazolam
Analgesics	Morphine Fentanyl
Paralytics	Succinylcholine Pancuronium Vecuronium Atracurium besylate Cisatracurium Rocuronium

M—*Medications/monitoring*: Medications already drawn up/cardiac monitor/blood pressure cuff/pulse oximetry
E—End-tidal CO_2 monitoring

■ INDUCTION AGENTS

- *Ketamine*:
    - *Dose*: 1.5 mg/kg IV, 4 mg/kg IM
    - Onset of action is around 60-90 seconds
    - *Duration*: 10-20 minutes
    - *Use*: Safe to use in prehospital conditions, especially in underlying reactive airway disease (asthma)
    - *Side-effects/drawbacks*: Use with caution with patients with significant cardiovascular comorbidities, as causes increase in sympathetic stimulation.
- *Thiopentone*:
    - *Dose*: 3-5 mg/kg IV
    - *Onset of action*: 30-45 seconds
    - *Duration*: 5-10 minutes
    - *Use*: Drug of choice in status epilepticus
    - *Side-effects/drawbacks*: Contraindication in patients with known porphyria, hypotension, and myocardial depression.
- *Propofol*:
    - Propofol 1-2.5 mg/kg
    - *Onset of action*: 15-45 seconds
    - One of the most commonly used induction agents, easy to use
    - *Duration*: 5-10 minutes
    - *Use*: Widely used in ED for RSI (in trauma/head injury/asthma/hemodynamically stable patients)
    - *Side-effects/drawbacks*: Pain on injection site and significant hypotension are the most common side-effects.
- *Midazolam*:
    - *Dose*: 0.3 mg/kg IV
    - *Onset of action*: 60-90 seconds
    - *Duration*: 15-30 minutes
    - *Use*: Not recommended for routine RSI, but can be useful in severe hemodynamically unstable patients
    - *Drawbacks*: Variable response with respiratory depression and paradoxical agitation.

- *Etomidate*:
  - *Dose*: 0.3 mg/kg IV
  - *Onset of action*: 10–15 seconds
  - *Use*: Widely used in ED for RSI for variety of conditions, use with caution with underlying sepsis
  - *Drawbacks*: Pain on injection site, significant adrenal suppression (debatable).

PARALYTIC AGENTS

- *Suxamethonium/succinylcholine*:
  - *Dose*: 1.5 mg/kg IV
  - *Onset of action*: 45–60 seconds
  - *Duration*: 6–10 minutes
  - *Use*: Widely used and quite safe to use
  - *Side-effects/drawbacks*: Hyperkalemia/bradycardia/significant fasciculations and is contraindicated in significant burns/malignant hyperthermia/crush injuries.
- *Rocuronium*:
  - *Dose*: 1.2 mg/kg IV
  - *Onset of action*: 60 seconds
  - *Use*: Widely used with no significant contraindications. Reversal agent is sugammadex
  - *Side-effects/drawbacks*: Anaphylaxis (rare).
- *Vecuronium*:
  - *Dose*: 0.15 mg/kg IV
  - *Onset*: 2–3 minutes
  - *Duration*: 45–60 minutes
  - *Use*: It should not be ideally used for RSI
  - *Drawbacks*: It has slow onset and long duration makes it not suitable for RSI in ED.

REFERENCES

1. Nickson C (2020). Sedation in ICU – LITFL. [online] Available from: https://litfl.com/sedation-in-icu/ [Last accessed February, 2021].
2. General anesthetics. In: Katzung & Trevor's Pharmacology Examination and Board Review, 9th edition. McGraw-Hill Companies, Incorporated; 2010.
3. Respiratory Therapy Zone (2020). Drugs Used in Mechanical Ventilation for Sedation and Pain Control. [online] Available from: https://www.respiratorytherapyzone.com/drugs-for-mechanical-ventilation/ [Last accessed February, 2021].

CHAPTER 7

Ventilatory Modes

■ INTRODUCTION

With the advent of mechanical ventilation, different modes of ventilation were introduced—each mode claiming a major advantage over other regarding improved ventilation, better gaseous exchange, less complications, morbidity and mortality, and reduction of work of breathing (WOB).

Instead, these modes have made positive-pressure ventilation more complicated and difficult to initiate.

Before proceeding with modes, let us look into the human respiratory cycle during mechanical ventilation.

Figure 1 focuses on the respiratory cycle on a ventilator.

Some terms are used for better understanding of the respiratory cycle on the ventilator:

- *Triggering*: It means change from expiration to inspiration in a ventilator. A ventilator-driven breath may be given irrespective of patient having efforts or not (sensors in the ventilator detect

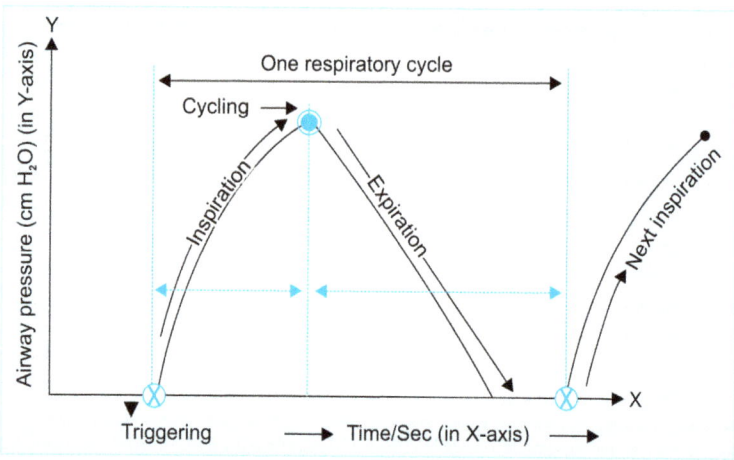

Fig. 1: Schematic diagram of respiratory cycle on a ventilator.

pressure or airflow changes that occur in ventilatory circuit, if the patient initiates any respiratory effort or does not have any). In other words, patient may or may not trigger the ventilator to get a mechanical inspiratory breath.
- *Cycling*: This means change over from inspiration to expiration.

Cycling has following determinants:
- *Volume cycle (basis of volume control ventilation)*: The inspiratory breath given by the ventilator is terminated after a specific volume has been delivered to the patient. Thereafter, expiration begins.
- *Flow cycle [basis of pressure support ventilation (PSV)]*: The machine cycles back to expiration once inspiratory flow has decreased to a certain level, e.g., either to a fraction of peak flow (usually 25% of peak inspiratory flow) or absolute value (e.g., 5 L/min).
- *Time cycle*: After a fixed time, the ventilator cycles to expiration when the preset inspiratory time in the ventilator is over.
- *Pressure cycle (basis of pressure controlled ventilation)*: After a fixed predesignated pressure level is reached as per ventilator settings, the ventilator cycles back to expiration.

All mechanisms of cycling in modern ventilators are either based on volume or pressure or on "*mixed*" cycling. Newer ventilators come with time cycling too.

CLASSIFICATION

The major modes of ventilation under discussion are as follows:
- Volume control mode
- Pressure control mode.

Volume Control Mode

- This is the most popular method as per the worldwide statistical figures.
- It uses a constant "*inflation volume*" for ventilation as per the need of the patient.

It can be subdivided into following modes as discussed here.

Control Mode Ventilation (CMV)

The ventilatory requirements of the patient are under complete control of the treating physician. All parameters are set on the ventilator and thoroughly monitored.

In such mode, generous use of sedatives and paralytics may be necessary.

This mode is appropriate for patients having no or little respiratory effort or under conditions where ventilatory parameter of the patient needs to be totally controlled by the physician.

The treating doctor sets the "*tidal volume*" and also "*respiratory rate*", as per the ventilatory requirements of patient.

Assist Mode

In this mode, ventilator gives a tidal volume (breath) when patient triggers it. Whenever the patient tries to breathe by himself, he triggers the ventilator into giving an inspiratory breath **(Fig. 2)**.

The patient is thus able to breathe at his own rate. In this mode, a fixed tidal volume is set and the patient determines the rate at which he breathes.

Since this mode does not have any "*back-up breaths*", the ventilator will not give a tidal volume unless triggered by the patient himself.

The deflection below baseline: (1) represents drop in airway pressure produced by effort of patient to initiate respiration (triggering); (2) is the positive breath given by the ventilator.

Assist Control Mode Ventilation

Newer ventilators come with this mode instead of pure "*Assist*" mode. In this mode, a "*backup*" rate is provided, which is set by the physician **(Fig. 3)**.

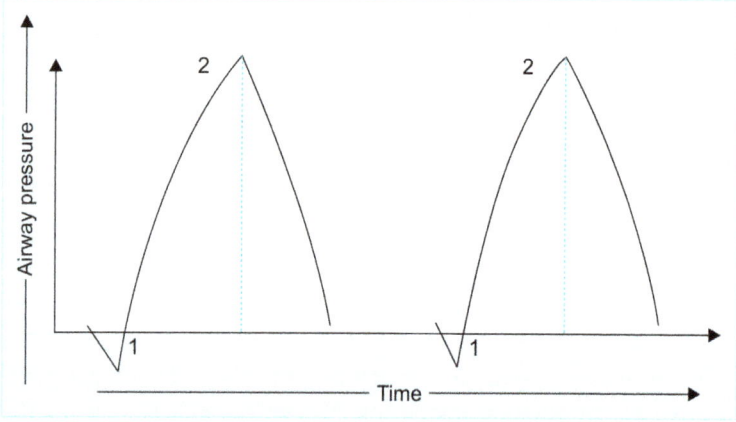

Fig. 2: Schematic presentation of assist mode.

CHAPTER 7 | Ventilatory Modes

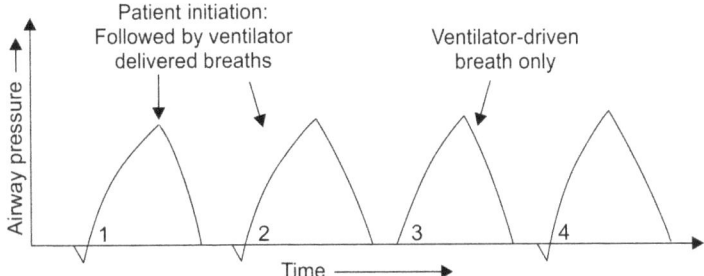

Fig. 3: Schematic presentation of assist control mode ventilation.

So, all patient initiated breaths (spontaneous) are delivered in "*Assist*" mode. However, if due to the diseased process, the patient is unable to initiate a breath, the ventilator ensures delivery of breaths at a minimum respiratory rate, set as a "*backup*" in the ventilator by the treating physician.

Now, consider the following settings in a ventilated patient in assist control mode ventilation (ACMV) mode.

Tidal volume (TV) = 450 mL and respiratory rate (RR) = 10 breaths/min.

Supposing, the patient is triggering the ventilator in this mode at 18 times per minute. So, the ventilator is giving him assisted breath of TV = 450 mL at the rate of 18 times a minute. This is assist mode (*pure assist*).

For some reasons, if the patient is not able to trigger the ventilator (may be due to deterioration of primary condition for which the patient was ventilated), this patient would still get assisted breaths at the rate of 10 times per minute set on ventilator with the same tidal volume in ACMV mode.

So, the ACMV guarantees minimum ventilatory requirements via a backup rate, while also allowing the patient to breathe spontaneously.

In **Figure 3**, 1, 2, and 4 are patient-triggered positive-pressure ventilatory breaths. The patient has failed to trigger the ventilator after second breath. So the ventilator delivers a breath by itself (3), which is a positive-pressure ventilatory breath without initiation or triggering.

A final word about ACMV:
- In this mode, WOB is performed mainly by the ventilator.
- Patient has to spend energy to "*trigger*" the ventilator.
- Patient's inspiratory effort does not cease, once ventilator is triggered.
- Proper inspiratory time should be set and matched with ventilator's inspiratory and expiratory cycle.

Intermittent Mandatory Ventilation (IMV)

This is primarily a weaning mode.

In this mode, mandatory (compulsory) breaths are given to the patient irrespective of the patient's own demands. In between mandatory breaths, the patient is free to breathe at his own respiratory rate.

The number of mandatory breaths per minute and also the tidal volume has to be set. The compulsory (mandatory) breaths are delivered at equal intervals of time, intermittently.

The tidal volume of spontaneous breaths will depend on patient's inspiratory effort strength. If a patient cannot generate a sufficient inspiratory force to create a satisfactory tidal volume during his spontaneous breath, alveolar hypoventilation will occur.

So, mandatory (compulsory) rate has to be set high to fulfill the ventilatory requirements of the patient **(Fig. 4)**.

The gentle undulations above baseline (in the diagram below) represent patient's spontaneous respirations. The mandatory vent-driven positive pressure breath is represented by (III).

Now, if any "*asynchrony*" occurs between the patient who is taking spontaneous respirations and the ventilator delivering

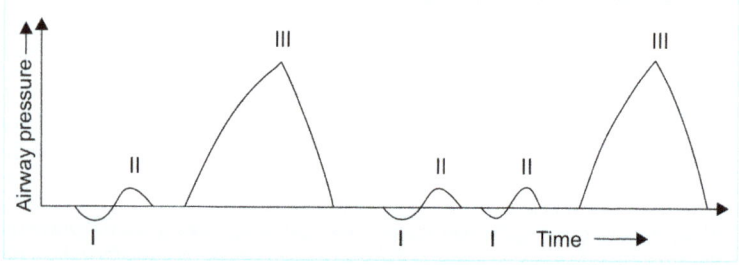

Fig. 4: Schematic representation of intermittent mandatory ventilation.

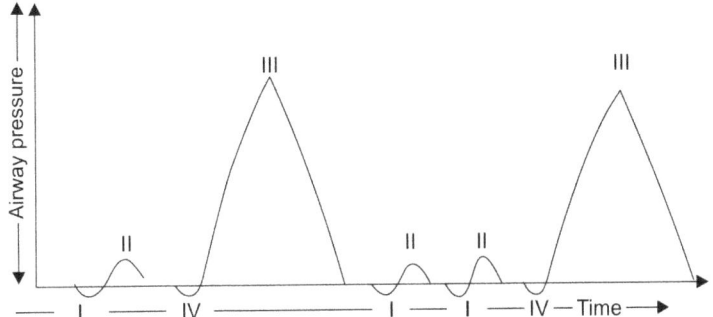

Fig. 5: Schematic representation of synchronized intermittent mandatory ventilation mode.

breaths; *"Clashing of Breaths"* occurs, which means patient and ventilator are in disharmony (also known as *"Breath Stacking"*).

In order to prevent this *"asynchrony"*, a newer mode was developed known as synchronized intermittent mandatory ventilation (SIMV).

Synchronized Intermittent Mandatory Ventilation

In this mode, the ventilator detects the onset of patient's spontaneous inspiratory efforts and delivers a mandatory breath in synchrony with the patient's spontaneous inspiration **(Fig. 5)**.

The mandatory (III) breath is synchronized with patient's spontaneous inspiratory effort (IV).

When SIMV mode is selected in a ventilator for a patient, an indicator is seen on ventilator's control panel indicating pressure support (PS) or PSV mode. What does it mean?

We have seen spontaneous breaths taken by a patient in SIMV mode in the below diagram. These spontaneous breaths are of very small tidal volume and they are not participating in any meaningful ventilation to help the patient.

In order to have a proper meaningful alveolar ventilation in such patients, the volume of these spontaneous breaths is boosted up by external PS, leading to combination of two modes (SIMV + PSV mode).

A final word about IMV/SIMV:
- IMV/SIMV is used principally as a weaning mode.

- Synchronized intermittent mandatory ventilation allows patient to use his own respiratory muscles by gradually transferring the ventilatory burden from the ventilator to the patient.
- Patient is free to increase or decrease his spontaneous respiratory rate and thus fulfill his ventilatory requirements.
- The generation of spontaneous breath in SIMV mode requires creation of negative intrathoracic pressure—similar to normal physiological respiration.

Pressure Support Ventilation

During PSV, the ventilator supports the inspiratory effort of patient with positive pressure. Expiration is as always passive **(Fig. 6)**.

Since the doctor sets the "*level*" of PS in the ventilator during inspiration, the levels of tidal volume can be made to rise and fall, in accordance to levels of variations of the PS.

In **Figure 6**, (I) represents airway pressure during unassisted breaths, and (II, III) represent varied airway pressure during pressure supported breaths.

With the onset of inspiration, airway pressure rises, maintains a plateau in inspiration and then decreases toward expiration, thus allowing expiration to occur passively.

"*Flow cycling*" is the norm of PSV. The flow threshold that determines cycling to expiration, from rise and plateau of inspiration,

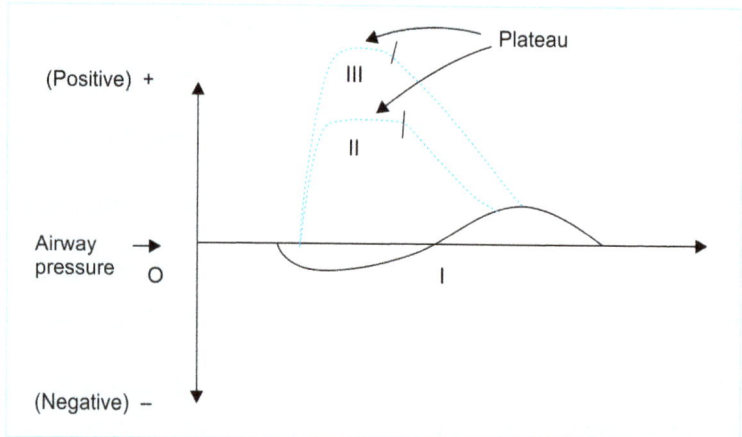

Fig. 6: Schematic representation of pressure support ventilation.

is generally 25–30% of peak flow for most of the ventilators, i.e., expiration occurs when airflow during phase of inspiration falls to 25–30% of its peak level. In addition to "*flow cycle*", PSV is also backed by addition of "*time cycle*" in some newer generation ventilators. The inspiratory breaths are automatically terminated after a certain inspiratory time has elapsed in such ventilators.

Criteria for PSV:
- Ideally, the patient must "*ask for*" a breath from ventilator by attempting to initiate a spontaneous respiration, which causes a dip in airway pressure (detected by ventilator's pressure change sensors).
- The patient must be able to trigger the ventilator on his own.
- Patient can control respiratory frequency and can breathe at respiratory rate he chooses of his own.
- The patient can control depth, length, and flow profile of each breaths.

A final word about PSV:
- Pressure support ventilation minimizes WOB.
- Pressure support ventilation decreases respiratory rate and increases tidal volume making breathing comfortable.
- Low level PS 5–10 cm H_2O can negate additional WOB that ET imposes (since lumen of ET is much smaller than "*innate*" airway).
- Maximum PS in many ventilators varies from 35 to 50 cm H_2O.

Continuous Positive Airway Pressure (CPAP)

This mode can be used in those patients who are breathing spontaneously (*a must*).

At the end of expiration, pressure in the airways equals to the pressure at mouth and both equate with normal atmospheric pressure. Surfactant prevents collapse of alveoli at this low end-expiratory pressure **(Fig. 7)**.

In diseased state, the alveoli collapse at low end-expiratory pressures due to lack of surfactant. So, hypoxia occurs as a result of V/Q mismatch and shunting occurs.

Large number of alveoli collapse during the disease process leading to decreased lung compliance. Higher inflation pressure is

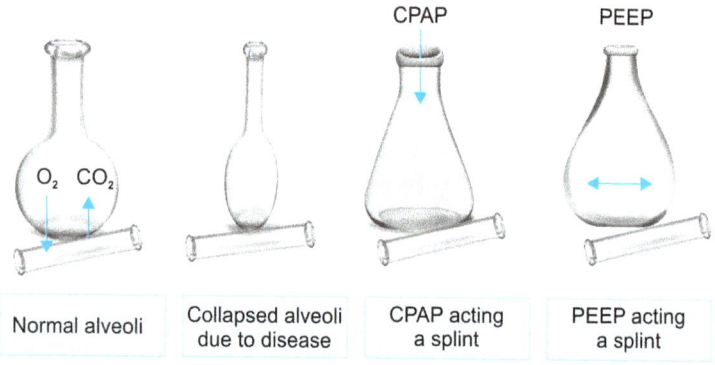

Fig. 7: Schematic diagram for CPAP. (CPAP: continuous positive airway pressure; PEEP: positive end-expiratory pressure).

then often needed to open or inflate the diseased alveoli. Once lung compliance decreases, more energy is needed to inflate the lungs, so "*WOB*" also increases.

Thus, high pressures needed to open alveoli may result in alveolar rupture leading to barotrauma.

Continuous positive airway pressure and positive end-expiratory pressure (PEEP) both act as "*internal splints*" for unstable collapsing alveolar units. CPAP also elevates end-expiratory pressure above atmospheric pressure, thus keeping unstable alveolar units from collapsing and thus participating in the "*recruitment*" of them for useful ventilation. CPAP helps in the recruitment of collapsed alveoli, thereby increasing functional residual capacity of the lung.

Continuous positive airway pressure also decreases the "*WOB*". CPAP can reverse hypoxia by restoration of ventilation to the perfused areas (recruitment), thereby improving lung compliance. Stabilization of upper airways is also an additional purpose of this mode.

Bilevel Positive Airway Pressure

Continuous positive airway pressure does not provide support during inspiration, as it only maintains positive pressure in airways. So, PSV was added to provide PS during inspiration in patients with poor respiratory effort. This resulted in creation of a new mode called bilevel positive airway pressure (BIPAP).

Bilevel positive airway pressure has two components:
1. Pressure support ventilation, which acts as inspiratory pressure.

2. Positive end-expiratory pressure, which acts as end expiratory pressure.

The BIPAP and CPAP both have disadvantage of propensity toward hyperinflation of lung.

Combining the modes discussed above, newer modes have been developed for better patient's ventilator management. All newer modes come with their own advantages and limitations.

Alternate modes of ventilation are also available, when conventional modes of ventilation are not sufficient for some patients with acute respiratory failure, where hypoxemia is refractory to oxygen therapy and conventional mechanical ventilation. These modes of ventilation are called *Rescue Modes of Ventilation*. High frequency oscillatory ventilation (HFOV) and airway pressure release ventilation (APRV) fall under the category of rescue mode of ventilation.

"Open Lung Concept" of mechanical ventilation is to open up the lung and keep the lung open. Consequently, the adverse effects of alveolar collapse can be mitigated by these modes of ventilation seen below.

Airway Pressure Release Ventilation

Generally, it uses prolong periods of spontaneous breathing at high end-expiratory pressures, which will be interrupted by brief periods of pressure release to atmospheric pressure. It is a variant of CPAP with an intermittent release phase. This mode is mainly used in patients with acute lung injury/acute respiratory distress syndrome (ALI/ARDS) where convention ventilatory management fails.

Airway pressure release ventilation can attain complete recruitment of diseased alveoli by maintaining high pressures over long durations resulting in better arteriolar oxygenation and lower peak pressures leading to less incidence of volutrauma **(Fig. 8)**.

High Frequency Oscillatory Ventilation

It uses high frequency, low volume oscillations leading to high mean airway pressure, which in turn leads to recruitment of diseased alveoli.

The low tidal volumes (1–2 mL/kg) prevent barotrauma.

High frequency oscillatory ventilation requires specialized ventilator, which allows control of frequency *(determined from*

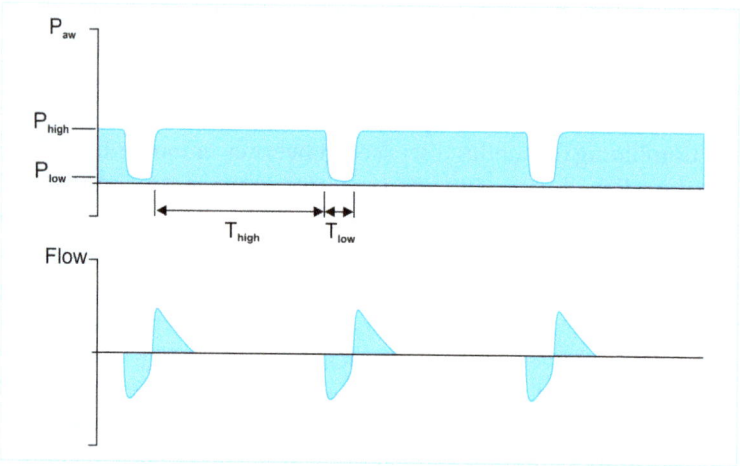

Fig. 8: Airway pressure release ventilation.

arterial pH) and amplitude of oscillations *(4-7 Hz is 240-420 oscillations)*, mean airway pressure *(set to 5 cm of H_2O above end inspiratory alveolar pressure during CMV)*, inspiratory time *(33% of respiratory cycle)*, and bias flow rate *(40 mL/min)*.

Finally to conclude, depending on the ventilatory requirements of the patients the treating physician has to choose the appropriate modes on the ventilator needed to manage the patient.

■ KEY POINTS

- Normal respiration starts with creation of a negative pressure inside the thoracic cavity. Inspiration is an active process, while expiration is passive. During inspiration, intrapulmonary pressure is generally negative.
- In absence of any respiratory effort by the patient or when paralytic drugs are used in the patient, ACMV mode becomes CMV mode.
- Application of PS increases tidal volume of spontaneous breaths only and not of mandatory breaths.
- So this mode will supposedly produce less hemodynamic instability in patient.
- CPAP/BIPAP can be used in both intubated and nonintubated patients via both invasive/noninvasive ventilators.

CHAPTER 8

Noninvasive Ventilation

NONINVASIVE VENTILATION OR NONINVASIVE POSITIVE-PRESSURE VENTILATION

In early 90s, increasing experience with positive-pressure ventilation led to development of a ventilatory strategy, where ventilation could be delivered through a well-fitted mask in patients of obstructive sleep apnea (OSA). Increasing success of noninvasive ventilation (NIV) in cases of OSA led to its adoption in ventilatory management of patients with chronic obstructive pulmonary disease (COPD). Finally, in the next ensuing 20 years, noninvasive positive-pressure ventilation (NPPV) delivered via a mask widely became adopted as the first-line ventilatory management in many medical centers over the whole world.

Noninvasive ventilation/NPPV refers to the administration of ventilatory support through the patient's upper airways using oronasal/nasal/similar masks without using an invasive artificial airway (endotracheal or tracheostomy tube). NIV has now become an integral tool in the management of both acute and chronic respiratory failure, in both hospital and home settings. NIV is being used as a replacement for invasive ventilation in many cases due to its advantages and flexibility.

The basic concept of NPPV is the application of positive pressure during the respiratory cycle (inspiration and expiration). The simplest application of that is a continuous positive pressure throughout the respiratory cycle, which is named CPAP (continuous positive airway pressure). The next application is administration of two different levels of pressure, one for inspiratory phase and one for the expiratory phase, otherwise known as BiPAP (bilevel positive airway pressure).

Noninvasive positive-pressure ventilation operates with application of positive pressure to upper airway (via interface/masks) either by using a conventional ventilator or specialized equipment like BiPAP/CPAP machines. NPPV can also be given by volume cycled or pressure cycled ventilators. CPAP/BiPAP/PSV (pressure support ventilation)/other modes can all be used in NIV, as per ventilatory needs of the patient.

How does NPPV Work?

Noninvasive positive-pressure works by:
- Decreasing inspiratory work of breathing (WOB)
- Decreasing inspiratory muscles work
- Decreasing "pressure time product" (PTP) of inspiratory muscle—an index for muscle O_2 consumption [PTP of diaphragm is reduced by 25% with PSV alone, while with PSV + PEEP (positive end-expiratory pressure), it goes down to 40%].

Interface

Interface or masks are devices, which connect ventilator tubings to facial region of the patient during NIV. Patient-ventilator interfaces available for NPPV include a full face mask/oronasal mask/nasal mask/nasal prongs/helmets. The full face mask includes the eyes, nose, and mouth, while the oronasal mask includes the nose and mouth, but not the eyes. A simple nasal mask is also available **(Fig. 1)**. Straps hold the interface in place and should be adjusted to avoid excess pressure on the nose or the face. The straps should be loose enough to allow one or two fingers to pass between the face and the strap. When a nasal mask is used, a chin strap is usually necessary to maintain closure of the mouth.

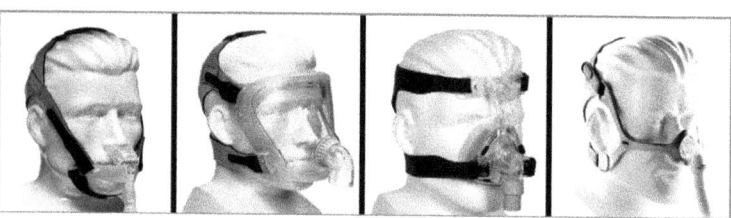

Fig. 1: Different types of interface attachments.

The efficacy of the various interfaces has been debated over years. The face mask confers physiologic improvement, but the nasal mask is better tolerated. Whichever mask is selected, it is helpful to keep the following points in mind:

- Most patients with acute respiratory failure are mouth breathers; therefore, NPPV delivered by a nasal mask may result in a larger air leak through the mouth, thus leading to a poor outcome.
- The nasal air passages offer significant resistance to airflow, which can reduce the beneficial effects of NPPV, if low positive pressure is used.
- The monitoring for aspiration in NPPV patients is often difficult.
- Humidification of the inspired air is difficult through any form of masks.

The helmet interface has been used to improve patient tolerance in many cases. Moreover, the helmet interface allows patients to talk, read, and drink through a straw, while minimizing complications such as skin necrosis, gastric distension, and eye irritation. But this interface may cause accumulation of CO_2 within the helmet, may produce noise sufficiently high enough to cause hearing damage, and may also to lead to more patient-ventilator asynchrony, and less relief of inspiratory effort of the patient.

What Type of Ventilators can be used for NPPV?

Noninvasive ventilation can be delivered via special type of noninvasive ventilators found in most emergency rooms/intensive care units (ICUs) of hospitals or by a portable normal invasive ventilator. Now a days "*Hybrid ventilators*" offering both forms (invasive and noninvasive) of ventilatory support are also available. However, the standard invasive ICU ventilator has numerous advantages over the BiPAP/CPAP machines. The advantages are:

- A precise concentration of oxygen can be delivered, i.e., FiO_2 can be set.
- Separate inspiratory and expiratory tubing minimizes the rebreathing of expiratory gases like carbon dioxide.
- Large mask leaks or patient's disconnection can be readily detected.
- Better monitoring and alarm features are present in standard ventilators.

- Higher inspiratory pressures (>20 cm H_2O) can be given if need arises.
- Backup ventilation is present when needed.
- In addition, certain modes can only be delivered by a standard ICU ventilator only (e.g., volume controlled, pressure controlled, time-limited PSV, etc.).

What Modes of Ventilator can be used for NIV?

The NPPV can be delivered using the same modes that are used for invasive mechanical ventilation, although certain modes may be used more frequently:
- *Assist control mode* is the most common mode chosen by doctors who want a specific amount of minute ventilation.
- *Pressure support ventilation* is the most common mode chosen by doctors who focuses on patient's comfort and synchrony.
- *CPAP/BiPAP* is used for patients with acute respiratory failure.
- *Proportional assist ventilation* delivers an inspiratory pressure that is proportional to patient effort. This allows better patient-ventilator synchrony.

How to Set the Ventilator for NPPV?

The selected mode in the ventilator automatically shows which parameters are need to be set during the initiation of NIV on the front/digital panel of the machine, e.g., assist control mode requires a tidal volume, respiratory rate, inspiratory flow rate, PEEP, and (FiO_2) to be set.

The BiPAP mode will show both inspiratory positive airway pressure (IPAP) and expiratory positive airway pressure (EPAP) settings, respiratory rate, PEEP, and other parameters if available.

Selection Criteria for NPPV

First and foremost criterion of selection is that, patient should be *conscious and spontaneously breathing.*

Patient should have the ability to protect airway himself, be co-operative and also should be hemodynamically stable. Care should be taken that there are no excessive respiratory secretions present in such patients, undergoing a trial of NPPV.

Selecting patients for NPPV requires careful consideration of its indications and contraindications. A trial of NPPV is worthwhile in most patients who do not require emergent intubation and have a disease known to respond to NPPV.

Conditions known to respond to NPPV are as follows:
- Exacerbations of CPOD where $paCO_2$ > 45 mm Hg or pH < 7.30
- Cardiogenic pulmonary edema
- Acute hypoxemic respiratory failure
- Obstructive sleep apnea–hypopnea syndrome
- Congestive heart failure
- Obesity hypoventilation syndrome
- Acute exacerbations of COPD
- Immunocompromised host with acute respiratory failure
- Postextubation and respiratory failure after extubation
- Facilitate weaning
- Asthma and status asthmaticus.

Contraindications for NPPV

The need for emergent intubation is an absolute contraindication to NPPV.

Noninvasive positive-pressure ventilation is also contraindicated in following conditions:
- Patients having no spontaneous breathing
- Unconscious patient
- Severe hemodynamic instability of the patient
- Upper airway obstruction
- Facial trauma in a patient
- Pneumothorax
- Inability to cooperate, protect the airway, or clear secretions
- High aspiration risk
- Prolonged duration of mechanical ventilation anticipated
- Recent esophageal anastomosis.

How to Initiate NPPV in Patients?

It should be done through graded steps which are as follows:
1. Selection of proper interface is foremost followed by acclimatization of the patient with the interface/mask.
2. Start with low pressure/volume in spontaneous mode.

3. O_2 supplementation should be continued @ 3-5 L/min and adjusted/increased as per need.
4. Initial IPAP should be started at 8-10 cm H_2O while EPAP at 3-4 cm H_2O.
5. An IPAP:EPAP ratio should be kept constant at 2.5:1.
6. Gradual increase of both pressures at 1-3 cm H_2O increments should be done.
7. Care should be taken that pressure should not exceed >20 cm H_2O.

Monitoring of Patients on NPPV

After NPPV is initiated, the patient should be observed closely for the first 4-6 hours to troubleshoot, provide reassurance, and look for deterioration of clinical condition of the patient. Improvement of the pH and arterial carbon dioxide tension ($paCO_2$) within one-and-a-half to two hours predicts better success rate.

In contrast, conditions like worsening encephalopathy or agitation, inability to clear secretions, inability to tolerate any of the interfaces, hemodynamic instability, or decreased oxygenation may indicate toward failure.

The use of sedatives and analgesics is sometimes employed by clinicians to increase tolerance and comfort of NPPV as well as to treat comorbid anxiety or pain.

Predictors of Success of NPPV

One of the most consistent signs of favorable response to NPPV is drop in respiratory rate within first to second hour of starting of NPPV.

The following parameters should be considered for successful NPPV trial:
- $paCO_2$ > 45 and <90 mm Hg at initiation of NPPV
- pH > 7.1 at initiation of NPPV
- Less air leakage via interface during NPPV
- Ability of the patient to coordinate breathing with the ventilator
- Lower severity of illness [APACHE (Acute Physiology and Chronic Health Evaluation) scores] and young age of the patient.

Weaning

Weaning from NPPV may be accomplished by progressively decreasing the amount of positive airway pressure, permitting the patient to be disconnected from the NPPV for progressively longer durations, or acombination of both.

Complications of NPPV

These are common complications:
- Leakage via mask leading to multiple adjustments
- Intolerance of positive pressure by patient
- Gastric distention due to positive pressure
- Aspiration (rare)
- Facial skin breakdown (long-term use)
- Increased gastric pressure may lead to abdominal compartment syndrome
- Hypotension
- Barotrauma.

■ KEY POINTS

Continuous Positive Airway Pressure

- This mode can be used in patients who are breathing spontaneously (a must). At end expiration, pressure in airways equals to pressure at mouth and both equate with normal atmospheric pressure. Surfactant prevents collapse of the alveoli which would have otherwise collapsed at this low end-expiratory pressure.
- In diseased state, the alveoli collapse at low end-expiratory pressures due to lack of surfactant. So, hypoxia occurs resulting in V/Q mismatch and shunting. Large number of alveoli collapses during disease process in lungs leading to decreased lung compliance. Once lung compliance decreases, more energy is needed to inflate the alveoli. So, higher inflation pressures are needed to open the diseased alveoli. Thus, "WOB" increases.
- Such high pressures needed to open diseased alveoli may also result in alveolar rupture leading to barotrauma.
- Continuous positive airway pressure and PEEP both thus act as "internal splints" for unstable alveolar units. CPAP also elevates

end-expiratory pressure above atmospheric pressure thus keeping unstable alveolar units from collapsing and then finally "recruiting" them for useful ventilation. CPAP also helps in the recruitment of collapsed alveoli thereby increasing functional residual capacity of lung.
- Continuous positive airway pressure thus decreases "WOB." CPAP can reverse hypoxia by restoration of ventilation to perfused areas (recruitment), thereby improving lung compliance. Stabilization of upper airways is also a purpose of this mode.

Bilevel Positive Airway Pressure

- Continuous positive airway pressure does not provide support during inspiration as it only maintains positive pressure in airways. So, PSV was added to provide pressure support during inspiration in patients with poor respiratory effort. This resulted in creation of a new mode called BiPAP.
- So, BiPAP has two components providing pressures at two levels, i.e., inspiratory and expiratory level:
    - Pressure support ventilation—which provides inspiratory pressure.
    - Positive end-expiratory pressure—which provides expiratory pressure.
- Bilevel positive airway pressure and CPAP both have disadvantage of propensity toward hyperinflation of lung.

CHAPTER 9
Inspiratory Pressures and Flow Profiles

■ INSPIRATORY PRESSURES

In **Figure 1,** we can see that when the ventilator delivers breath, airway pressure rises gradually and progressively to peak inspiratory pressure, which is reached at end inspiration.

Thus, P_{peak} is sum of pressures required to overcome "airway resistance" and also the pressure required to overcome elastic properties of lung and chest wall. P_{peak} is also known as *Peak airway pressure.*

Now at the end of inspiration, if a hold is applied (usually an inspiratory hold *knob* in ventilator), no air or gas movement occurs inside the ventilatory circuit and the pressure drops to a certain level, called *Plateau inspiratory pressure* (P_{plat}). This P_{plat} reflects the pressure required only to overcome elastic recoil of lung and chest wall.

Plateau inspiratory pressure is the best indicator of peak alveolar pressure, which is an important indicator of alveolar distention. P_{plat} should always be maintained below 30 cm H_2O.

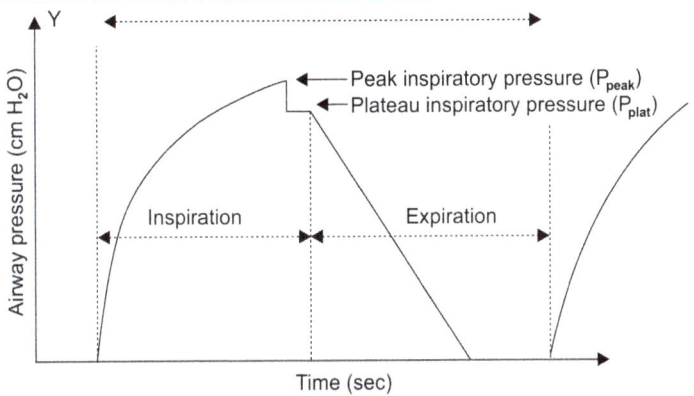

Fig. 1: Schematic diagram of peak inspiratory pressure.

Plateau inspiratory pressure can be reduced by: (1) decreasing tidal volumes (TV) and (2) by decreasing the positive end-expiratory pressure (PEEP).

As inspiratory pressure rises above normal limits, adverse effects like *barotrauma* (pneumothorax, pneumomediastinum) and *volutrauma* (alveolar surface rupture, parenchymal injury) can occur.

A final word about inspiratory pressures:
- These injuries (barotrauma, volutrauma) though linked with P_{peak}, correlate better with P_{plat}.
- Care should be taken about ventilator-induced lung injury (*VILI*).

■ FLOW PROFILES

Flow is defined as volume per unit time. The inspiratory flow can be profiled as per need of the patient to achieve varied clinical goals. The different types of flow can be classified into several waveforms:
- The square waveform
- The decelerating waveform
- The accelerating waveform
- The sine waveform.

The Square Waveform

When the inspiratory flow is constant and not varying through the delivery of tidal volume, the flow pattern is referred as square/rectilinear waveform. In this pattern, the inspiratory flow rises rapidly to certain level. The rate of flow is then held constant, until the set tidal volume has been delivered. The inspiratory flow rate often tends to decelerate toward the end of inspiration **(Fig. 2)**.

The Decelerating Waveform

It is also called reverse ramp flow pattern, as the inspiratory flow rate progressively decreases as inspiratory tidal volume is delivered. With this flow pattern, lung inflation with inspired tidal volume is slowed down toward the end of inspiration. As per theory, this pattern has advantage of reducing airway pressure. It is mainly used in "*pressure control*" modes **(Fig. 3)**.

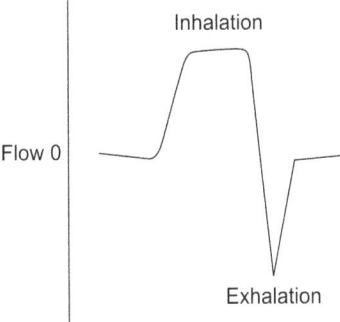

Fig. 2: The square waveform. The inspiratory flow rate remains uniform for the entire duration of the inspiratory breath.

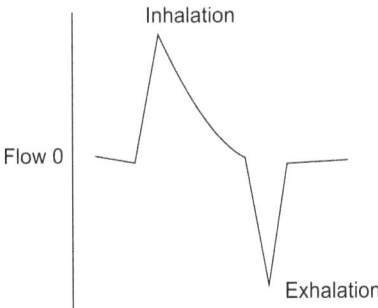

Fig. 3: The decelerating waveform. The inspiratory flow rate progressively slows down as the tidal volume is delivered to the patient.

The Accelerating Waveform

In this pattern, there is progressive increase in the rate of airflow with inspiration. At a set pressure, the airflow plateaus to rectilinear form and consistency in the flow rate is maintained till end of inspiration **(Fig. 4)**.

The Sine Waveform

In this waveform, the inspiratory flow increases to peak and then decreases again toward the end of tidal breath **(Fig. 5)**.

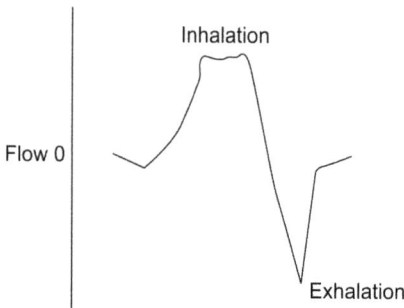

Fig. 4: The accelerating waveform.

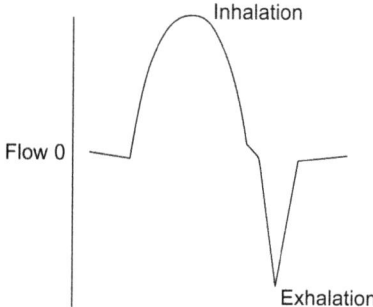

Fig. 5: The sinusoidal waveform. The inspiratory flow rate rises to a peak toward the middle of the inspiratory phase and then falls.

Volume control modes offer a better choice in terms of flow wave patterns.

CHAPTER 10

Pressure-Controlled Ventilation

■ INTRODUCTION

Pressure-controlled ventilation (PCV) is another mode of ventilation used in many patients. PCV mode allows more variation when patient's efforts and respiratory system impedance are poor.

A certain pressure is set in the ventilator during inspiration. During ventilator-driven breath/inspiration, pressure inside the airway rises as air is being pushed into the lungs. At a certain point, this airway pressure equates to the "pressure" set already on the ventilator. So, the ventilator delivers the breath maintaining this pressure for a duration of "set" inspiratory time (Ti/T insp.) **(Fig. 1)**.

So, "*pressure limit*" and "*fixed inspiratory time*" has to be set on the ventilator for this mode.

By varying the pressure limit, we can further vary the tidal volume (VT). Thus, higher pressure limit will increase VT and vice versa.

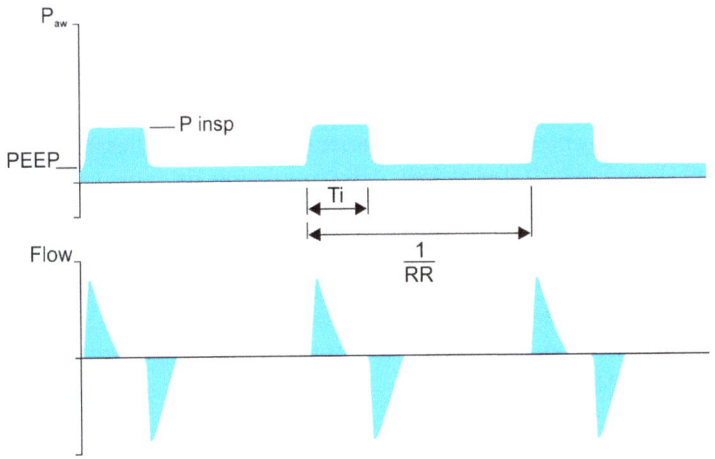

Fig. 1: Schematic presentation of pressure-controlled ventilation. (PEEP: positive end-expiratory pressure; P_{aw}: airway pressure; RR: respiratory rate; Ti: inspiratory time)

In this mode, "pressure limit" is generally set at ≤ 30 cm H_2O above positive end-expiratory pressure (PEEP). In addition, by fixing proper I:E ratio and respiratory rate (RR), inspiratory time can also be fixed.

It has to be remembered that "trigger sensitivity" should generally be kept low for proper triggering in PCV.

■ PRESSURE-CONTROLLED VENTILATION

During PCV, two pressure levels are kept constant: the lower pressure level PEEP and the upper pressure level (P insp). The volume and the decelerating flow are the resulting variables and can vary depending on changes in the lung mechanics.

The value controlled and kept at target value, by the equipment is the *pressures P insp*. The pressures PEEP and the number of mandatory breaths per minute (RR) can be adjusted. The difference between the two pressure levels *PEEP* and *P insp.*, the breathing effort of the patient, and the lung mechanics determine the breathing volume (VT) to be supplied. The minute volume (mV) can vary. With the slope adjustment, the pressure increase can be set to the upper pressure level depending on the patient.

A breath delivered by the machine can be divided into an inspiratory and expiratory phase. The duration of the inspiratory phase is defined by the inspiration time. During PCV, the upper pressure level is maintained for the duration of (Ti). The time for the next mandatory breath results from the number of mandatory breaths set in the ventilator (RR) and Ti.

If the lung mechanics of the patient and with it the Resistance (R) and Compliance (C) vary during the ventilation, this only influences the applied VT. The pressures remain constant. The pressures are also maintained in case of leakage.

Pressure control ventilation can be delivered in the following modes just like volume control ventilation:
- Pressure-controlled-continuous mandatory ventilation (*PC-CMV*).
- Pressure-controlled-assist control ventilation (*PC-AC*).
- Pressure-controlled-synchronous intermittent mandatory ventilation (*PC-SIMV*).
- Pressure-controlled-biphasic positive airway pressure (*BiPAP*).

CHAPTER 10 | Pressure-Controlled Ventilation

- Pressure-controlled–airway pressure release ventilation (*PC-APRV*).
- Pressure-controlled–pressure support ventilation (*PC-PSV*).

Volume guarantee: It ensures that for all mandatory breaths, the set *VT* is applied with necessary minimum pressure. If resistance and compliance of the lung changes, the pressure adapts gradually in order to administer the *VT*. Spontaneous breathing is possible during the whole breathing cycle.

PC-CMV: The VT supplied to the patient depends on pressure difference between *PEEP* and *P insp*. The number of breaths to be delivered is set by frequency (*RR*). The mandatory breaths are always machine triggered (*see* **Fig. 1**).

PC-AC: In this mode, if the patient attempts to breathe by himself, the breathing attempt at PEEP level triggers a mandatory breath from the machine. The patient thus determines number of additional mandatory breaths to be given by the ventilator. If the patient fails to trigger the machine, the machine will provide a compulsory breath (assist) as set by frequency (RR). So the machine assures a minimum number of compulsory breaths, if the patient fails to breathe by himself.

Also, sufficient time elapses before the patient is again able to trigger, thus giving sufficient time for expiration and completing the respiratory cycle **(Fig. 2)**.

PC-SIMV: In this mode mandatory breaths are synchronized with patient's own breathing attempts. Patient-triggered mandatory breaths can be triggered within a trigger window. This adaptation prevents a change in number of breaths (*RR*). In this mode, patient can breathe spontaneously during complete respiratory cycle. During spontaneous breathing at PEEP level, the patient's breath can be supported also by using pressure support (PS) **(Fig. 3)**.

PC-BiPAP: In this mode, patient can breathe spontaneously at any time, but number of mandatory breaths is specified. Mandatory breaths are synchronized in both inspiration and expiration. If mandatory breath is shortened on account of synchronization with expiration, the next breath is extended. Synchronization with inspiration shortens expiratory phase. Patient is free to breathe spontaneously during complete respiratory cycle **(Fig. 4)**.

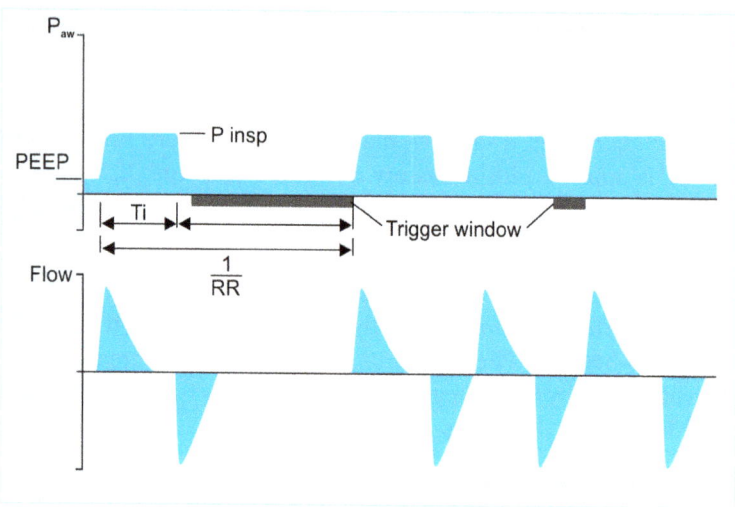

Fig. 2: Pressure-controlled–assist control ventilation.
(PEEP: positive end-expiratory pressure; RR: respiratory rate;
Ti: inspiratory time; P_{aw}: airway pressure)

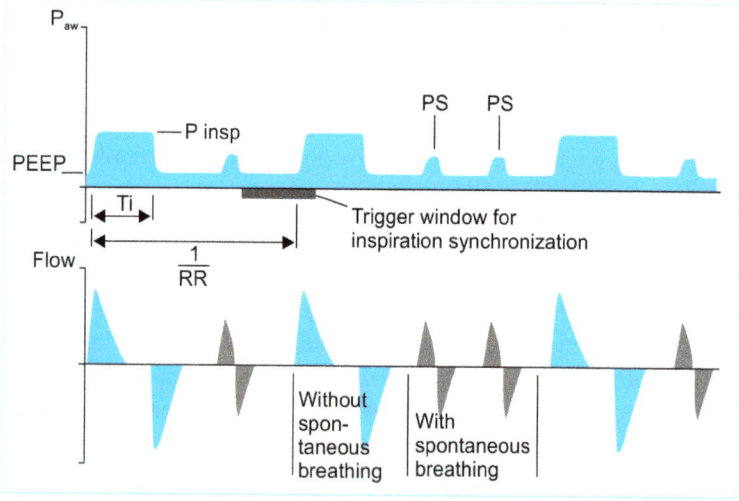

Fig. 3: Pressure-controlled–synchronous intermittent mandatory ventilation.
(PEEP: positive end-expiratory pressure; RR: respiratory rate;
Ti: inspiratory time; P_{aw}: airway pressure; PS: pressure support)

PC–APRV: In this mode, patient's spontaneous breathing takes place at upper pressure level P_{high}. This pressure level P_{high} is maintained for duration of T_{high}. For active expiration to happen, the pressure is reduced for a brief period T_{low} to P_{low}.

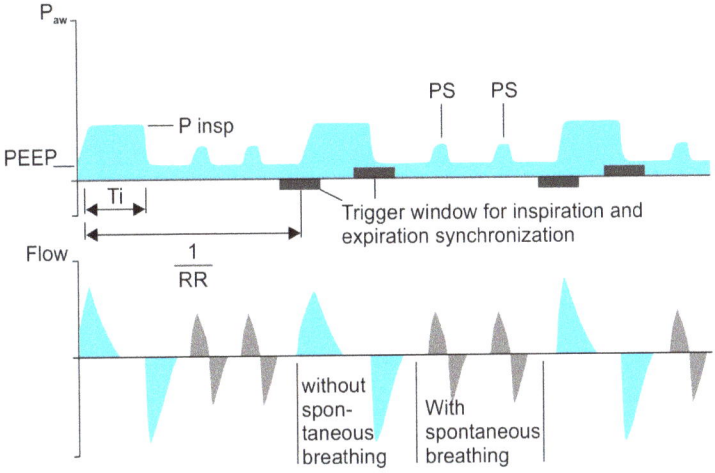

Fig. 4: Pressure-controlled–biphasic positive airway pressure. (PEEP: positive end-expiratory pressure; RR: respiratory rate; Ti: inspiratory time; P_{aw}: airway pressure; PS: pressure support)

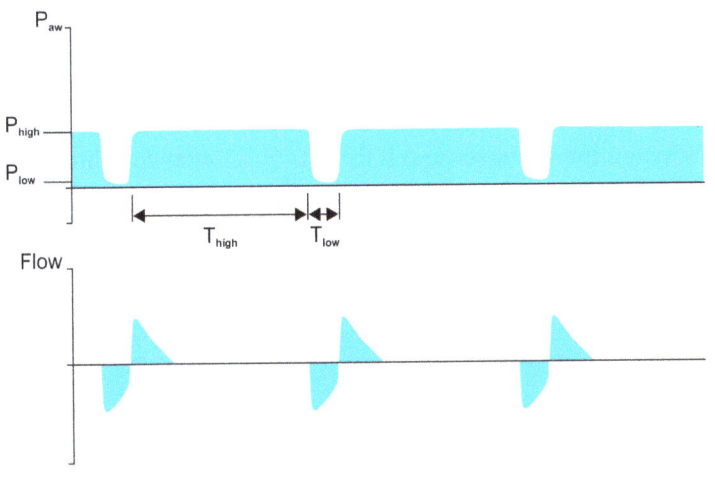

Fig. 5: Pressure-controlled–airway pressure release ventilation. (P_{aw}: airway pressure)

Also to help CO_2 elimination, the pressure is reduced to P_{low} for a brief period T_{low}. The alternation between these pressure levels is machine triggered and time cycled. The breathing volume (VT) expired is generated due to the above pressure differences **(Fig. 5)**.

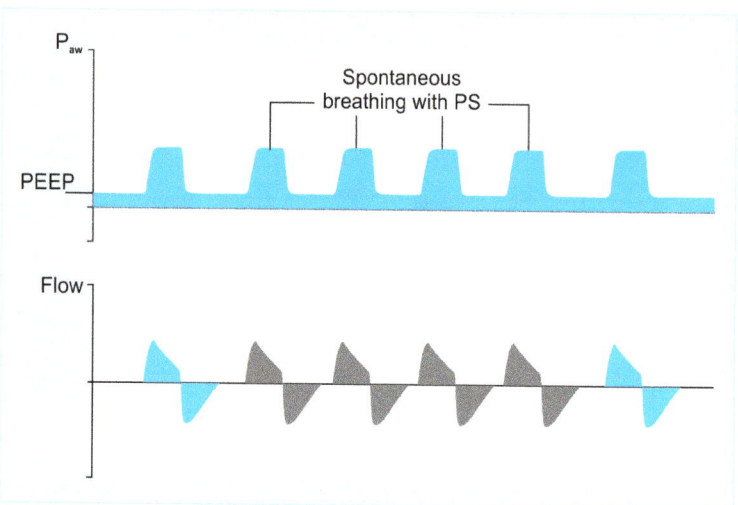

Fig. 6: Pressure-controlled–pressure support ventilation.
(PEEP: positive end-expiratory pressure; P_{aw}: airway pressure; PS: pressure support)

PC–PSV: In this mode, the patient can breathe spontaneously at *PEEP* level. Every detected inspiration effort is pressure supported. The duration of inspiration is flow cycled **(Fig. 6)**.

If the breathing frequency of the patient is lower than the backup rate set on the ventilator and if there is no spontaneous breathing, the patient will receive mandatory breaths with set pressure *P insp*.

The VT results from the pressure difference between *PEEP* and *P insp*.

CHAPTER 11

Positive End-Expiratory Pressure

INTRODUCTION

In a normal lung, ventilation throughout the lung is never uniform. In the upper parts of lung, due to higher negative pressures, the alveolar units become more distended at end expiration than the units in lower part of lungs.

Normal alveoli do not close completely even at very end of expiration. This is due to their *"surfactant"* content and also due to some amount of positive pressure in end of expiration (pressures generated by normal glottis) **(Fig. 1)**.

The positive end-expiratory pressure (PEEP) also serves as a *"splint"* for unstable or diseased alveoli, thus, preventing collapse during disease process.

In an intubated patient, glottic function is lost. To compensate for this loss, a small amount of PEEP is given in the ventilator in the range of 3–5 cm of H_2O which is known as *"Physiological PEEP."*

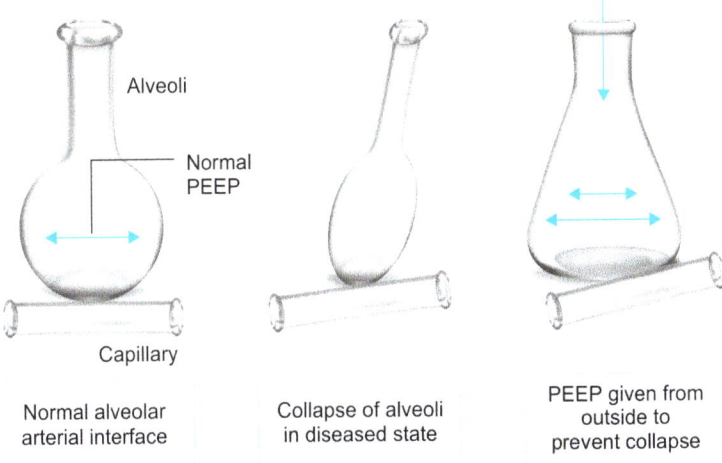

Fig. 1: Positive end-expiratory pressure (PEEP).

This level can "theoretically" prevent alveolar collapse that might occur in absence of functioning glottis.

The PEEP helps in tissue oxygenation by opening of collapsed alveoli, thereby increasing functional residual capacity (FRC) and thus decreasing shunt fraction by alveolar recruitment.

The PEEP, when used in higher levels, can have adverse effects on (1) oxygenation, (2) hemodynamic parameters, and (3) compliance of lungs.

Ideally, PEEP should be set in such levels that the lung operates on "steep" middle part of pressure-volume curve when lung mechanics and compliance are favorable (*see* Chapter 3 for pressure volume curve) **(Fig. 2)**.

Less than optimum PEEP causes lung to operate on lower parts of "pressure-volume curve" while high levels of PEEP cause lungs to function on higher parts of curve.

The PEEP should be given in "graded increments" and compliance should be calculated after every change in levels of PEEP.

Increased levels of PEEP elevate airway pressures producing alveolar over-distention and barotrauma. This alveolar distention causes compression of surrounding vessels thereby causing decreased venous return to heart, leading to hypotension. This effect is more profoundly seen in hypovolemic patients.

■ AUTO-PEEP

The respiratory cycle starts from initiation of one breath till initiation of next breath.

The respiratory cycle time is calculated by dividing 60 seconds (1 minute) by respiratory rate.

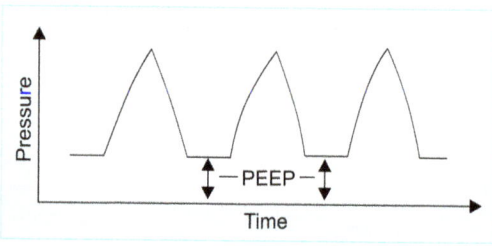

Fig. 2: Pressure-volume curve set by positive end-expiratory pressure (PEEP).

The ratio between the time spent on inhalation (*Inspiratory Time*) and on exhalation (*Expiratory Time*) constitutes I:E ratio.

During normal breathing, I:E ratio ranges between 1:1.5 and 1:2. The expiratory time is almost twice as long as inspiratory time.

In chronic lung diseases, expiration time becomes more prolonged and I:E ratio can increase up to 1:3, 1:3.5, or even more. Since expiration is always passive, expiration time is also thus passively determined.

If expiration time is too short, the previously ventilator-driven inspiratory breath cannot be completely exhaled. As a result, the next inspiratory breath given by the ventilator is superimposed on the residual gas of previous breath inside the lungs (generated due to incomplete expiration in the previous breath).

So, *breath stacking or clashing of breaths* occurs resulting in hyperinflation of lungs and development of additional PEEP (above the preset level of PEEP already set on the ventilator).

This increase in end-expiratory pressure is called "Auto-PEEP."

Auto-PEEP can be easily diagnosed from ventilatory graphics by viewing flow versus time graph **(Fig. 3)**.

The potential harmful effects of Auto-PEEP are same as those of higher levels of PEEP.

Auto-PEEP can be reduced by:
- Decreasing respiratory rate—fewer inspirations/minute.
- Decreasing tidal volume— small breaths need less time to deliver and less volume to exhale.

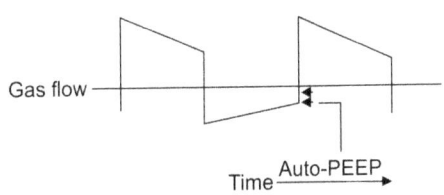

Fig. 3: Auto-PEEP is shown by failure of expiratory flow to return to zero before inspiratory flow is initiated.
(PEEP: positive end-expiratory pressure)

- Increasing gas flow rate—delivering tidal volume faster leading to more time for expiration.

A final word about PEEP:
- PEEP and auto-PEEP are mainly responsible for ventilator-induced lung injury (VILI).
- Judicious use of PEEP should be done.

◼ KEY POINT

Target of oxygenation of blood is to keep paO_2 > 60 mm Hg (confirmation by arterial blood gas). Trying to increase oxygenation above this level will not serve to increase O_2 delivery to tissues, since hemoglobin gets completely saturated at this level. So, this target paO_2 should be reached with as low as possible FiO_2. Higher levels of FiO_2 worsen lung injury. O_2 is itself toxic in higher concentrations.

CHAPTER 12
General Settings in a Ventilator

■ TIDAL VOLUME

This is the amount of air moving in and out of lungs with each breath. It should be optimized to the size of patient's lung.

Height is an important predictor for a tidal volume (TV) of a patient. However, in emergency room/ICU scenario, height is difficult to measure, so weight is taken as a surrogate for lung size—ideal body weight is taken rather than actual weight of patient.

	Ideal body weight calculation
Men	50 + 2.3 (height in inches—60)
	50 + 0.91 (height in cm—152)
Women	45.5 + 2.3 (height in inches—60)
	45.5 + 0.91 (height in cm—152)

Tidal volume can be used in ranges 5-8 mL/kg, as low TV ventilation is now the norm of the day, to prevent alveolar distention and injury associated with higher tidal TV (10-12 mL/kg).

■ RESPIRATORY RATE

Stable adult patients require 8-12 breaths/min. The respiratory rate (RR) should be ideally set as close to the normal rate.

Respiratory rate along with TV forms minute ventilation (MV) of a patient. So, variation of RR along with TV can be done to satisfy the patient's MV.

Higher RR will shorten respiratory cycle as a whole, thus decreasing both inspiratory and expiratory times.

In many ventilators, RR is directly related to inspiratory:expiratory (I:E) ratio parameter changes.

Hypercapnia and hypoxia also influence settings of RR in a ventilator greatly.

■ MINUTE VENTILATION

Normal MV is approximately 7–8 L/min.

Tidal volume × RR constitutes MV.

Tidal volume is also directly proportional to MV. So, any increase in TV will increase MV; leading to lowering of $paCO_2$ and vice versa.

Since MV = TV × RR, therefore alternating RR can also alter the levels of $paCO_2$.

Minute ventilation also correlates roughly with alveolar ventilation ($paCO_2$ is determined by alveolar ventilation), which is calculated as:

$$[V_A = (V_T - V_D) \times F]$$

where, V_D represents dead space and F is RR.

Thus, increase in MV (by increasing TV or RR) leads to fall in $paCO_2$ and vice versa.

■ FRACTION OF INSPIRED OXYGEN

When initiating ventilatory support, fraction of inspired oxygen (FiO_2) of 1.0 is used to ensure maximum amounts of available O_2 during resuscitation, followed by patient's adjustment to ventilator and to stabilize the patient's oxygen requirements. Goal of treatment should be to bring FiO_2 levels to minimum (<40%) to maintain saturation more than 92% and above.

In addition, higher levels of FiO_2 are always a precursor for complication of oxygen therapy.

■ POSITIVE END-EXPIRATORY PRESSURE

For positive end-expiratory pressure (PEEP) details, *see* Chapter 10: Pressure-controlled Ventilation.

■ INSPIRATION-EXPIRATION TIME RATIO

The "*respiratory cycle time*" is calculated by dividing 60 seconds (1 minute), by RR. Normal physiological I:E ratio varies between 1:1.5 and 1:2.

Now consider a patient is in a ventilator, having parameters like RR = 10 breaths/min and I:E ratio of 1:2. Respiratory cycle time will be calculated by dividing 60 seconds (1 minute) by RR.

Therefore, 1 minute = 60 s/10 = 6 seconds (total respiratory cycle time).

So, as per I:E ratio of 1:2, out of 6 seconds above, 2 seconds are spent in inspiration and 4 seconds in expiration (2 + 4 = 6 = total respiratory cycle time in seconds).

The I:E ratio is directly related to RR. Higher RR will cause shortening of I:E ratio leading to air trapping inside the lungs.

When inspiratory time is prolonged or equal to the length of expiratory time (e.g., I:E = 1:1 or 2:2 or 2:1), the physiological I:E is said to be *inverted*.

Inverse ratio ventilation (*IRV*) appears to increase oxygenation, which is mainly due to prolongation of inspiratory time, which affects mean airway pressures. IRV is uncomfortable and needs sedation and paralysis. IRV increases air trapping leading to barotrauma.

■ FLOW RATE

The flow rate during inspiration should be set to match patient's demands.

Inspiratory flow needs to be set in range of (40–100 L/min). Several flow rate patterns are seen like rectilinear, accelerating, decelerating, sinusoidal, etc.

A slow flow rate results in lower inspiratory time. On other hand, increasing inspiratory flow rate will increase peak airway pressure, leading to barotrauma.

■ SLOPE

It adjusts how quickly the higher pressure level is reached. The P *insp* is maintained for duration of *Ti*.

■ TRIGGER SENSITIVITY

Trigger sensitivity is the negative pressure, the patient has to create (since normal respiration initiates with negative pressure in thoracic cavity), which the ventilator pressure sensors need to detect before delivering tidal breath. This detection is done by pressure/flow transducers of the ventilator.

The purpose is to coordinate delivery of inspiratory breath by ventilator, synchronously with patient's own inspiratory effort.

Trigger sensitivity should be kept low, so that patient spends minimum energy to trigger the ventilator but not so low, that spontaneous triggering of the ventilator happens by miniscule pressure changes, which normally occurs inside the ventilatory circuit during functioning of the ventilator.

Appropriate trigger sensitivity would range between −0.5 and −1.5 cm H_2O.

■ INSPIRATORY PEAK/PLATEAU PRESSURE

For ventilator pressure details, *see* Chapter 8: Noninvasive Ventilation.

■ SETTINGS OF VENTILATOR AS PER MODE SELECTION

The following settings are generally seen in volume control modes. When volume control mode is selected, the following parameters may be seen on the ventilator control panel **(Fig. 1)**. Some ventilators may show less/more settings on the panel as different modes are selected like VC–AC (volume-controlled–assist control ventilation), VC-SIMV (volume controlled–synchronous intermittent mandatory ventilation), etc.

Similarly in pressure control mode, the following settings in the machine are seen as per selection of different pressure control modes **(Figs. 2A to C)**. So, there may be increased or decreased number of settings on the control panel as per selection of pressure control modes, e.g., PC-AC (pressure-controlled–assist control ventilation), PC-SIMV (pressure-controlled–synchronous intermittent mandatory ventilation), PC-APRV (pressure-controlled–airway pressure release ventilation), etc.

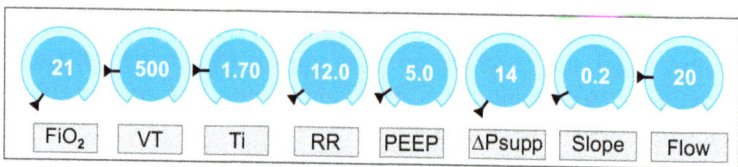

Fig. 1: Volume control mode. (VT: tidal volume; Ti: inspiratory time; RR: respirator rate; PEEP: positive end-expiratory pressure; Psupp: pressure support)

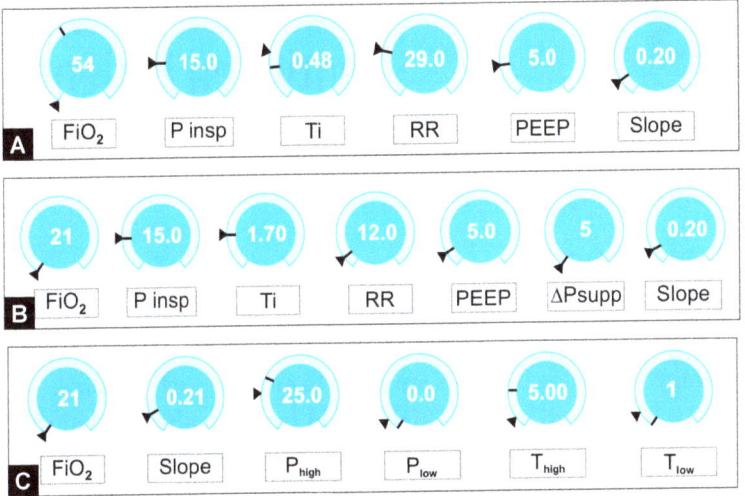

Figs. 2A to C: Pressure control mode.
(Ti: inspiratory time; RR: respirator rate; PEEP: positive end-expiratory pressure; Psupp: pressure support)

Ventilator Settings for Better Oxygenation

It can be done by:
- Increasing FiO_2
- Increasing alveolar ventilation (*increasing MV by changing TV or RR*)
- Judicious use of PEEP.

This can also be done by:
- Inverse ratio ventilation
- Prone ventilation
- Increasing O_2 carrying capacity of blood: correcting anemia/heart failure.

■ KEY POINTS

FiO_2 in normal atmosphere can be expressed as 0.21 or 21%. Any supplemental O_2 above atmospheric levels increases O_2 percentage by 4% every liter of O_2.
   Therefore,
- L/minute O_2 = 25% (21% + 4%) of FiO_2
- L/minute O_2 = 29% of FiO_2 L/minute O_2 = 33% of FiO_2 and so on.

CHAPTER 13

Monitoring of Ventilated Patients

INTRODUCTION

Patients on ventilatory support require continuous monitoring to assess beneficial and adverse effects of this form of supportive therapy. The following steps are taken to monitor such patients:
- Arterial blood gases (ABG) should be done after initiation of mechanical ventilation and then intermittently, based on clinical status of the patients.
- Arterial blood gas will provide valuable information of oxygenation (paO_2), ventilation ($paCO_2$), and acid-base balance (pH). Assessing paO_2 and pH together and setting the ventilator accordingly, is a necessity.
- A proper clinical assessment of the patient should be done and hemodynamic parameters should be strictly monitored.
- Pulse oximetry must be done regularly to monitor oxygenation and proper corrections of oxygenations should be made accordingly.
- Chest radiographs are to be obtained after intubation and additional chest X-rays are done for assessing the condition of patient on regular basis.
- A "track" of inspiratory plateau pressures (via ventilator control panel) and a watch on pressure alarms should be kept.
- *Capnography*: By providing a real-time estimate of $paCO_2$, capnography measures alveolar ventilation, respiratory gas exchange, and CO_2 production. It also helps in assessing return of spontaneous circulation (ROSC) during cardiopulmonary resuscitation (CPR).

Normal $PETCO_2$ ranges between 35 and 45 mm Hg **(Fig. 1)**.

Phase I: It represents low CO_2 tension in the gas expelled from the anatomical dead space.

CHAPTER 13 | Monitoring of Ventilated Patients

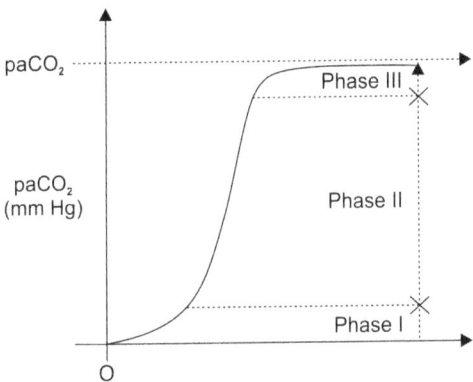

Fig. 1: Capnography.

Phase II: It represents increasing CO_2 tension as exhaled gases come more from the alveolus.

Phase III: It represents CO_2 plateau, since exhaled gases are mainly from the alveoli.

VENTILATOR ALARMS

Ventilator alarms are also used to monitor and alert caregivers about abnormal ventilatory parameters seen in the patients after initiation of ventilation:
- *Low pressure alarms* start when there is a:
  - Leakage in the ventilatory circuit
  - Ventilator disconnected from the patient
  - ET tube cuff rupture or leakage.
- *High pressure alarms*: This alarm is generally set 10 cm H_2O above the baseline peak airway pressure of the patient. High pressure alarms get activated when there is:
  - ET tube obstruction or kinking
  - Excess secretions blocking ET
  - Bronchoconstriction
  - When lung compliance decreases in conditions like:
    - Pneumothorax
    - Pulmonary edema

- Biting of ET tube by patient, immediately after intubation and in absence of maintenance of proper sedation and paralysis.
- *Apnea alarm* is activated when there is no inspiratory effort from patient's side for at least 10–20 seconds in a spontaneous mode of breathing [e.g., bilevel positive airway pressure (BiPAP) and synchronized intermittent mandatory ventilation (SIMV)].
- *Low FiO_2 alarm*: If FiO_2 levels fall below FiO_2 levels set in the ventilator, this alarm will be activated. It is mainly due to decrease in O_2 concentration in the piped wall supply unit of the hospital.
- *High FiO_2 alarm*: Will be activated if there is a drop in central piped air supply—since proportion of O_2 raises in the gas mixture coming via piped unit, which supplies a mixture of oxygen and air.

Ventilatory Complications in Emergency Room

CHAPTER 14

VENTILATORY COMPLICATIONS

The following complications are common in the emergency room during intubation and initiation of ventilation:

- *Right bronchus intubation*: Since the right bronchus is more aligned with trachea, a deep endotracheal tube (ET) will enter the right bronchus more often. This results in blockage of left bronchus by ET resulting in lack of aeration and collapse of left lung. Thereby the tidal volume intended for both lungs goes to one, resulting in adverse effects of "volutrauma."
  To avoid this complication, ET should be fixed properly with tapes/ET fixators/bandage rolls (common practice). Studies show ET moves substantially with flexion and extension of neck. Studies also show ET tube fixators prevent less movement of ET than other methods.
  Ideally, ET should be fixed at 23 cm in men and 21 cm in women from incisors of the patient and should be at least 2-4 cm above the carina. The position of ET should be checked with radiographs of chest-particularly after intubation and after adjustments of tube position.
- *Endotracheal tube obstruction*: It generally occurs insidiously but may be liable to sudden obstruction, as secretion gradually builds up. The lumen may be narrowed by encrustations or a sudden clot or a plug of sputum may suddenly lodge and block the entire diameter of the tube. Proper suctioning goes a long way to prevent such complication. Further change of ET may be considered in such cases.
- *Endotracheal tube migration*: ET may actually migrate downward with flexion of neck and vice versa. It may migrate in either of the bronchus. So, proper fixation of ET is necessary.
- *Endotracheal tube cuff leak*: A sudden ability of an intubated patient to *vocalize* may point toward a cuff leak. Pooled secretions

above the cuff may tickle down to lower airways after leak and can increase the risk of ventilator-associated pneumonia (VAP). A sudden loss of airway pressure may also point toward cuff leak (low pressure alarm kicks in).

- *Self-extubation*: This can lead to catastrophic results. A self-extubation by an unstable patient may be due to pain/disorientation/asynchrony between the patient and the ventilator.

  It can be prevented by deep sedation, paralytics, and restrainment.

- *Bronchospasm*: It can occur in hyper reactive airways due to irritation of airways by ET. Nebulization via ET can prevents as such complications.

- *Laryngeal/pharyngeal/tooth trauma*: It can occur and should be managed in standard lines.

- *Arrhythmias*: Various arrhythmias may occur, seen more commonly in young adults and children. About 4% of patients suffer cardiac arrest during intubation and ventilation.

  Arrhythmias should be managed as per advanced cardiac life support (ACLS) protocols:

- *Tracheostomy complications*:
  - Complications in previously tracheostomized patients coming to emergency room
  - Emergency room physicians often have to deal with patients having previous tracheostomy. Common complications encountered in such patients are as follows:
    - Blockage of tube and cuff leaks
    - Tracheoesophageal fistula—due to ischemic necrosis of tracheal mucosa by high cuff pressure
    - Tracheoinnominate artery fistula (rare)—pressure producing necrosis of tracheal wall with erosion of the artery
    - Tracheocutaneous fistula.

Proper care and gentle handling during changing of tube, and proper cuff pressure helps in preventing such complications.

■ KEY POINT

An imaginary position of carina can be assessed by the meeting point of two imaginary straight lines drawn on chest radiograph. One imaginary straight line is drawn through center of trachea and the other one is drawn through the middle of aortic knuckle.

CHAPTER 15: Ventilator-Induced Lung Injury and Ventilator-Associated Pneumonia

■ VENTILATOR-INDUCED LUNG INJURY

Barotrauma

Since ventilatory breaths are positive pressure breaths (external pressure is used to push breath), it will increase intrathoracic pressure. Increased intrathoracic pressure will raise alveolar pressure, which may lead to rupture of diseased alveoli.

Once alveolar rupture occurs—air tracks in mediastinum producing "pneumomediastinum." Mediastinal pleura eventually ruptures producing "pneumothorax."

Air from "pneumomediastinum" can dissect subcutaneous tissues of neck producing "subcutaneous emphysema." If air dissects down to peritoneum, "pneumoperitoneum" can also occur.

Other complications are "tension lung cysts" and systemic gas embolization.

Volutrauma

Alveolar overdistension can cause "pulmonary edema," "increased endothelial permeability," and "diffuse alveolar damage" leading to a condition, indistinguishable from acute respiratory distress syndrome (ARDS).

■ VENTILATOR-ASSOCIATED PNEUMONIA

Ventilator-associated pneumonia (VAP) is a pneumonia that develops 48 hours or longer after mechanical ventilation is initiated via endotracheal (ET) or after tracheostomy.

The diagnostic triad of VAP consists of following clinical criteria:
- *Pulmonary infection*: Signs include fever >38.3°C, purulent secretions and leukocytosis >12 × 10^9/mL.

- Bacteriological evidence of pulmonary infection.
- Radiological suggestion of pulmonary infection.

Two clinical criteria with combinations of radiological infiltrates increase sensitivity and specificity of VAP by 69% and 75%, respectively.

Organisms mainly suspected are multidrug-resistant (MDR) pathogens like *Enterobacter, Staphylococcus, Acinetobacter, Pseudomonas, Klebsiella,* and Enterobacteriaceae.

Scoring Systems for Ventilator-associated Pneumonia

To make diagnosis of VAP, some scoring systems are routinely used, although how much they help in diagnosis remains debatable:

- The CPIS score, also known as clinical pulmonary infection score, takes help of biomarkers like CRP and procalcitonin, though they have low predictive values **(Table 1)**.
- Centre of disease control and prevention has proposed ventilator-associated events (VAEs) definitions for epidemiological purposes of VAP **(Table 2)**.
- The 2016 IDSA-ATS (Infectious Diseases Society of America/American Thoracic Society)-VAP management guidelines suggested and recommended that only clinical criteria should be

TABLE 1: The modified CPIS.

CPIS points	0	1	2
Tracheal secretions	Rare	Abundant	Abundant + purulent
Chest X-ray infiltrates	No infiltrate	Diffused	Localized
Temperature (°C)	≥36.5 and ≤38.4	≥38.5 and ≤38.9	≥39 or ≤36
Leukocytes count (per mm³)	≥4,000 and ≤11,000	<4,000 or >11,000	<4,000 or >11,000 + band forms ≥500
PaO_2/FiO_2 (mm Hg)	>240 or ARDS		≤240 and no evidence of ARDS
Microbiology	Negative		Positive

(ARDS: acute respiratory distress syndrome; CPIS: clinical pulmonary infection score).
Source: Produced with permission from American Thoracic Society guideline.

TABLE 2: The ventilator-associated events.

Ventilator-associated complication (VAC)	At least one of the following indicators of worsening oxygenation following a sustained period of stability or improvement on the ventilator for ≥2 calendar days: • Minimal daily FiO_2 values increase ≥0.20 (20 points) over baseline and remain at or above that increased level for ≥2 calendar days • Minimum daily PEEP values increase ≥3 cm H_2O over baseline or above that increased level for ≥2 calendar days
Infection-related ventilator-associated complication (IVAC)	Patient has VAC and also fits both of the two following criteria: • Temperature greater than 38°C • Or WBC > 12,000 or <4,000/mm³ • A new antimicrobial agent is started and is continued for 4 or more calendar days
Possible VAP	Patients with IVAC and one of the following criteria is met: • Gram stain evidence of purulent respiratory secretions • Positive respiratory culture
Probable VAP	Patients with IVAC and Gram stain evidence of purulent respiratory secretions plus quantitative or semiqualitative growth of a pathogenic organism beyond specified thresholds for ET aspirate: 10^6, bronchoscopic or mini BAL 10^5, PSB 10^3, or positive diagnostic test for *Legionella spp.*, or positive diagnostic test on respiratory secretions for influenza virus, respiratory syncytial virus, adenovirus, parainfluenza virus

(BAL: bronchoalveolar lavage; ET: endotracheal tube; PEEP: positive end-expiratory pressure; PSB: protected specimen brush; VAP: ventilator-associated pneumonia)
Source: Produced with permission from American Thoracic Society guideline.

used for diagnosis of VAP and no scores with biomarkers should be used.

As per IDSA–ATS guidelines management of VAP is as given in **Flowchart 1**.

Flowchart 1: Guidelines for management of ventilator-associated pneumonia (VAP).

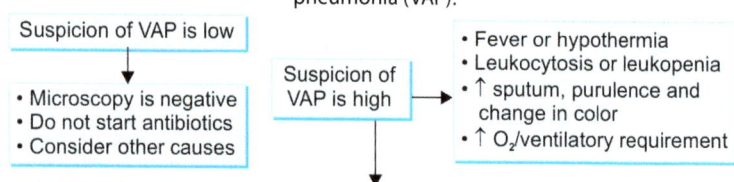

Suspicion of VAP is low
- Microscopy is negative
- Do not start antibiotics
- Consider other causes

Suspicion of VAP is high
- Fever or hypothermia
- Leukocytosis or leukopenia
- ↑ sputum, purulence and change in color
- ↑ O_2/ventilatory requirement

Send the following:
- Paired blood culture
- Noninvasive endotracheal aspirate (double catheter blind technique or invasive LRTI sample (BAL, PSB)
- Other relevant cultures
- *Biomarkers*: CRP, serum procalcitonin
- Look for risk factors for MDR

Start empiric antibiotic therapy that covers for *S. aureus, Pseudomonas aeruginosa* and other relevant GNB's (avoid colistin, it other effective agents are available):
- Therapy should cover for MRSA with Linezolid or vancomycin, if MRSA risk is high
- If no MRSA risk is present, therapy should cover for MSSA
- If initial choice is piperacillin-tazobactam, cefepime, levofloxacin, imipenem, meropenem, do not add specific MSSA agents like oxacillin, nafcillin or cefazolin

After the culture reports are available:
- If bug is sensitive only to polymyxins or aminoglycosides → Use IV + inhaled therapy
- If bug is resistant to carbapenems, use IV polymyxins + inhaled colistin
- De- escalate to specific antibiotics if pathogen identified
- Stop antibiotics if culture is sterile and patient is clinically improved
- Antibiotic therapy should be stopped after 7 days
- A longer therapy may be considered, if clinical, radiological signs are still unresolved and laboratory parameters are not improved

Specific antibiotic therapy:
Acinetobacter:
- If isolate is susceptible, use carbapenem, ampi-sulbactam, pip-tazo
- It sensitive only to polymyxin, use IV polymyxin and inhaled colistin
- Do not use rifampicin or tigecycline

Pseudomonas:
- Avoid aminoglycosides
- Use one antibiotic, if no risk factors are present for antimicrobial resistance
- Use two antibiotics from different class, if risk factors for antimicrobial resistance are present

(BAL: bronchoalveolar lavage; CRP: C-reactive protein; IV: intravenous; LRTI: lower respiratory tract infection; MDR: multidrug resistant; MRSA: methicillin-resistant *Staphylococcus aureus*; MSSA: methicillin-sensitive *S. aureus*; PSB: protected specimen brush)

Prevention of Ventilator-associated Pneumonia

Prevention of VAP is shown in **Table 3**.

TABLE 3: Prevention of ventilator-associated pneumonia.

Pharmacological methods	Nonpharmacological methods
Hand hygiene with alcohol based solution	Use of noninvasive mask ventilation
Oral care with chlorhexidine	Avoid reintubation
Short course of antibiotic therapy (when clinically applicable)	Orotracheal and orogastric intubation
• Sedation control and weaning protocol • Manage without sedation whenever possible/interupt sedation daily	Use of heat moisture exchanger
Restricted blood transfusion	Closed endotracheal suction
Vaccines (influenza and pneumococcal)	Subglottic secretion drainage
Prophylactic probiotic	Automated control of endotracheal tube cuff pressure
	Mechanical tooth brushing
	Ultrathin polyurethane endotracheal tube cuff
	Saline installation before endotracheal suctioning
	Change of ventilator circuit only for each new patient
	Semirecumbent positioning (elevate head end of bed 30–45°)
	Shortening duration of mechanical ventilation (assess readiness to extubate daily/perform spontaneous breathing trials with sedatives turned off/facilitate early mobility)
	Adequate intensive care staffing
	Use of protocol bundles
	Education and training

Source: Produced with permission from American Thoracic Society guideline.

CHAPTER 16: Weaning Parameters

INTRODUCTION

Weaning means gradual decrease of mechanical ventilatory support in a graded manner, so as to prepare the patient for spontaneous respiration of his own.

It should be considered as soon as the patients have recovered sufficiently from the ongoing illness. Other prerequisites include "preserved sensorium" and stable "cardiovascular parameters."

Several criteria must be checked before weaning:
- Metabolic alkalosis—depresses respiratory drive—should be corrected.
- Gastric distention—hampers diaphragm movement—correction should be done.
- Sedatives are to be stopped—depress respiratory centers.
- Paralytic agents/aminoglycosides should be stopped—act on neuromuscular junctions preventing optimal respiratory muscle contraction.
- An elevated "respiratory rate" with "tachycardia" must be looked for; these are early signs of failure of weaning.
- Use of accessory muscles of respiration is a sign of increased work of breathing.
- Hemoglobin levels should be checked.

There are also several weaning parameters like:
- Oxygenation/ventilation parameters
- Respiratory muscle strength parameters
- Respiratory muscle endurance parameters
- Inspiratory load parameters.

Except the oxygenation parameters, other parameters are not to be assessed in the emergency department.

Ideally, weaning parameters should be assessed by an intensivist in an ICU. Emergency physicians practically have no role in weaning process.

PREREQUISITES FOR WEANING

- Patient's present disease condition should be improving.
- Hemodynamic stability should be assessed and all vasopressors should be stopped.
- Oxygenation parameters should be adequate. ($PaO_2/FiO_2 > 300$, positive end-expiratory pressure (PEEP) < 5 cm of H_2O, SpO_2 > 90% with $FiO_2 < 40\%$).
- Patient must have spontaneous inspiratory efforts of his own.
- Patient should be afebrile, mentation normal, should have normal hemoglobin status, and stable metabolic status.
- The Rapid Shallow Breathing Index (RSBI) is most accepted weaning predictor. RSBI is assessed by putting patient on T piece for 2 minutes. *F/TV < 100 is a predictor for successful weaning* (F = frequency, TV = tidal volume).
- Minute ventilation < 10 L/min.
- Respiratory rate (RR) <10 >35 breaths/min.
- Diaphragm incursions and excursions during respiration and diaphragmatic thickening fractions assessed by ultrasound are promising new weaning parameters.

After stoppage of all sedatives in such patients, a trial of spontaneous awakening should be done (*SAT*). Now if the patient is fine with *SAT*, above prerequisites have to be taken into account and a trial of spontaneous breathing (*SBT*) should be started.

Spontaneous Breathing Trial (SBT) can be done as follows:
- *T-piece*: It is connected to endotracheal tube (ET)/tracheostomy tube and the patient is made to breathe humidified oxygen-air mixture for 30-120 minutes. SBT should be done once in 24 hours. Repeated T piece trial in 24 hours does not help much.
- *Pressure support*: It is maintained at 6-8 cm of H_2O and PEEP of 4 cm of H_2O. It is gradually reduced, titrated, and patients comfort is seen.
- If successful, extubation can be tried after reassessing the patient again and also care should be taken to look for postextubation failure which may be evident again by rising heart rate (HR)/RR/$paCO_2$ and falling oxygen saturations.

CHAPTER 17

Ventilatory Strategies

■ INTRODUCTION

Emergency physicians commonly have to face medical emergencies, which need ventilatory support. A guideline for proper ventilatory management of these conditions has been highlighted in this chapter.

■ CHRONIC OBSTRUCTIVE LUNG DISEASE/ASTHMA

Ventilate such patients with:

- *Low tidal volume (TV)* (5–8 mL/kg), i.e., lung protective ventilation.
- *Rate* (10–12 breaths/min) as per need of the patient, thus satisfying his/her ventilatory demands. Care should be taken that backup rate is not very low. Ideally to begin with, respiratory rate (RR) should be kept between 8 and 12 breaths/min. Rate can be increased once there is a need to bring down $paCO_2$. However, rate should not exceed >20 breaths/min.
- *High inspiratory flow rate* (60–80 L/min) allows more complete lung emptying thus decreasing plateau pressure.
- *I:E ratio* should be set carefully to begin with; normal ratio of 1:1.5 to 1:2 should be kept. Once there is an evidence of air trapping, I:E ratio can be increased (1:3) at least to allow more time for expiration.
- *Positive end-expiratory pressure (PEEP)* should be set to ≤5 cm H_2O to avoid over inflation.
- *Plateau pressure* should be kept below 30 cm of H_2O.
- *Peak pressures* may be often generally high >60 cm of H_2O and may increase with higher flow rate.
- Vigilant care toward air trapping and dynamic hyperinflation (which may result in *auto-PEEP*) is recommended.
- Avoid *dynamic hyperinflation* by keeping inspiratory time short, avoiding inspiratory pause, increasing inspiratory flow rate,

square form of flow delivery, and decreasing TV and minute volume leading to *permissive hypercapnia*.
- Care should be taken to switch the patient from assist control modes to spontaneous modes.
- Patients are very much prone to respiratory muscle exhaustion due to increased work of breathing due to narrowed airways. Therefore, weaning should be difficult in such patients. Ideally, noninvasive positive pressure ventilation (NIPV) trial should be given first, if it is not contraindicated in such patients.
- *Awake intubations* (sedatives + opioids for pain management) and plus-minus paralytics should be considered.
- *Heat* and *moisture exchangers* should not be used in ventilator circuit. *Nebulizers* should be used in inspiratory tubing of ventilator 30 cm before universal connector.

FLAIL CHEST

- *Normal ventilation with proper PEEP can act as a splint for flail segment, which collapses during inspiration.* PEEP should be kept minimum between 5 and 8 cm of H_2O.
- Flail chest is responsible for decrease in vital capacity and producing a stiff lung. The reduced functional residual capacity (FRC) due to flail segment causes respiratory failure.
- *Bilevel positive airway pressure (BiPAP) or continuous positive airway pressure (CPAP) has been beneficial in such cases.* These modes help in splinting the flail segment by pressure support. These modes can also be applied by invasive ventilators in major traumas.
- In less severe trauma, noninvasive ventilation might help, and a trial of NIPV can be started and observed.

HEAD INJURY

- *Normal ventilatory strategy* (*normal standard settings*) to maintain normal $paCO_2$ levels. All normal parameters are set in the ventilator.
- *Protection of airway*: Poor Glasgow Coma Scale (GCS) may lead to aspiration, so protection of airway is paramount.
- *Hyperventilation is not recommended*: Normal ventilation rule is keeping $paCO_2$ levels near normal or slightly lower than normal levels.

- *Prevention of intracranial pressure (ICP) rise*: Agitation/fighting the tube/restlessness/excessive movements/distended bladder can increase ICP. So, paralytics can be considered for first 12 hours, and then gradually withdrawn.

NEUROMUSCULAR DISEASES (GUILLAIN-BARRÉ SYNDROME/MYASTHENIA GRAVIS/AMYOTROPHIC LATERAL SCLEROSIS/MYASTHENIA GRAVIS/POLIOMYELITIS)

- Problems with *respiratory muscles mainly*. May exhibit type II respiratory failure.
- Respiratory center and its neural inputs are normal.

Since respiratory drive is normal, *normal settings on the ventilator may be with a* higher *TV* can be considered. All ventilator parameters are kept as close to normal. These patients tend to develop atelectasis when adequate TVs are not given. Caution should be taken regarding use of paralytics, during intubation and later periods of ventilation due to actions of such drugs on neuromuscular junctions.

MYOCARDIAL INFARCTION/HEART FAILURES/HYPOVOLEMIC SHOCK

- Since normal heart is preload dependent, care should be taken about venous return. Avoid excessive pressures.
- Balance between oxygenation by positive pressure and normal cardiac output should be maintained and monitored.
- *High ventilatory pressure [mainly pressure control (PC)-pressure support ventilation (PSV) mode and pressures > 20 cm H_2O]* can predispose myocardium to ischemia.
- *Hypocapnia* promotes increased myocardial contractility and increased systemic vascular resistance, angina, and arrhythmias.

So aims in such above cases are as follows:
- Proper oxygenation [focus on normal FiO_2/minute volume (MV)/TV]
- Normal/near normal $paCO_2$ (normal frequency or RR)
- Ventilation (invasive/noninvasive) at lower pressures.

Care should be taken regarding increased PEEP, which has propensity to produce hypotension, by decreasing venous return to heart.

ACUTE RESPIRATORY DISTRESS SYNDROME

The following strategies may be considered in acute respiratory distress syndrome (ARDS):
- The main aim is to reverse hypoxemia and decrease work of breathing.
- Adequate monitoring is needed to prevent hemodynamic instability.
- Avoidance of barotrauma/volutrauma and prevention of ventilator-associated pneumonia (VAP) should be in the first priority list.
- In ARDS, lung should be considered as "baby lung," as it becomes stiff and also "sponge lungs" as dependent portions become more atelectatic. So, appropriate ventilatory measures are needed to recruit these portions of lungs for gaseous exchange.

Goals of mechanical ventilation in ARDS:
- Maintain paO_2 between 55 and 80 mm Hg and SaO_2 88–94%
- Plateau pressure <30 cm H_2O
- Driving pressure <14 cm H_2O
- pH to be maintained between 7.2 and 7.45 (permissive hypercapnia).

Settings: Either a volume control or a pressure control mode can be selected. Ideal body weight (IBW) has to be calculated. All patients should be administered neuromuscular agents for first 48 hours:
- Low TV ventilation (300–400 mL). TV 8 mL/kg IBW.
- Inspiratory pressure (Pplat) should be kept below 30 cm H_2O.
- Inspiratory flow or inspiratory time or I:E ratio time can be increased to increase oxygenation. A goal of I:E ratio should be maintained as close to 1:1.0–1.3.
- FiO_2 should be kept high initially and PEEP between 5 and 10 cm H_2O. Judicious use of PEEP and gradual increment of PEEP have to be done to maintain oxygenation. FiO_2 titration down to lower levels and application of increased levels of PEEP are done to maintain oxygen saturation above 90%.
- Incremental FiO_2–PEEP combinations to achieve oxygenation goal:

FiO_2	0.3	0.4	0.4	0.5	0.5	0.6	0.7	0.7
PEEP	5	5	8	8	10	10	10	12
FiO_2	0.7	0.8	0.9	0.9	0.9	1.0	1.0	1.0
PEEP	14	14	14	16	18	20	22	24

- Minute ventilation should be maintained as per patient's demand by varying RR (not to exceed >35 breaths/min).
- Monitoring and target goals of ventilation are to be achieved by manipulating the above parameters. While doing so if Pplat is rising >30 cm of H_2O, TV should be decreased by 1 mL/kg. But if asynchrony or breath stacking occurs, TV may be raised by 1 mL/kg keeping in mind platforms <30 cm of H_2O.
- pH goal to be maintained between 7.3 and 7.45. If pH is going down increase RR till pH is 7.3 or $paCO_2$ <25 mm Hg. By trying to do so if RR exceeds 35 and $paCO_2$ becomes <25 mm Hg, use bicarbonate infusions. Also TV can be increased to raise the pH.

■ RECRUITMENT STEPS

Method 1: Keep the patient in CPAP mode and deliver 40 cm H_2O pressure for up to 30s at FiO_2 of 1.0.

Method 2:
- Put patient in pressure control mode
- FiO_2 of 1.0
- Inspiratory pressure 40-50 cm H_2O
- PEEP 20-30 cm H_2O
- Rate 8-20/min
- Inspiratory time 1-3s
- Duration 1-2 min
- Start with lower inspiratory pressure (40) and PEEP (20) and if there is no response go to higher pressure.

Inverse ratio ventilation (IRV): When inspiration time in I:E ratio becomes equal to or greater than expiration time, ventilation is considered to be inverse. In IRV more time is given for inspiration in order to increase oxygenation. As a result, expiration is shortened leading to air trapping. This sort of ventilation is uncomfortable to the patient and needs proper sedation and paralytics. IRV depends on the "time constants" of lungs.

Prone ventilation increases FRC and oxygenation since most of pulmonary parenchyma is located posteriorly; gravitational changes due to prone position help in movement of water/secretions from large areas of lungs improving oxygenation. About 60–80% show appreciable reduction in their oxygen requirements with prone positioning. It reduces dorsal-ventral transpulmonary pressure difference and improves V/Q mismatch and bronchial drainage.

Prone ventilation is indicated when $paO_2/FiO_2 < 150$ with PEEP > 10 needed to maintain oxygenation. Each prone session should be of 18–24 hours duration and can be stopped if there is hemodynamic instability, no improvement of oxygenation after 4 hours of prone ventilation or worsening oxygenation. Ventilatory parameters would remain the same for ARDS treatment lines.

Permissive hypercapnia allows gradual rise of CO_2 by limiting minute ventilation so as to prevent inordinate elevation in the airway pressures.

If CO_2 is allowed to rise suddenly in blood (acute hypercapnia) the following complications may arise:
- Severe acidemia
- Arrhythmias
- Increase in ICP
- Increased levels of catecholamines increasing myocardial excitability
- Diminished renal blood flow
- Gastrointestinal bleed.

However, these acute problems do not occur, when CO_2 is allowed to rise in a slow and controlled manner, called permissivehypercapnia.

Permissive hypercapnia is used as a ventilator strategy in different diseased conditions needing ventilator support, when a steady and slow raise of $paCO_2$ is allowed, to maintain oxygenation of the patient.

Permissive hypercapnia is absolutely contraindicated in these conditions mentioned below:
- Cerebrovascular accident
- Epilepsy
- Coronary artery disease
- Cardiac arrhythmias
- Pulmonary arterial hypertension.

KEY POINTS

- Hypercapnia (increased $paCO_2$) causes cerebral vasodilation and further increases ICP.
- Hypocapnia (decreased $paCO_2$) causes cerebral vasoconstriction, which worsens cerebral ischemia.
- Hypocapnia also produces alkalosis and shifting of O_2 dissociation curve to left which impairs oxygenation of cerebral tissues.
- Now if $paCO_2$ is allowed to rise above normal levels, a rebound increase of ICP will occur with increased risk of reperfusion injury or hemorrhage to already ischemic penumbric regions of traumatized brain.

18. Ventilatory Graphics

INTRODUCTION

Ventilator graphics are essential tools in managing patient on ventilator. These graphics are generally displayed in two forms—scalar graphics and loops graphics.

Scalar graphs are generally expressed with these parameter relationships given below **(Fig. 1)**:
- Flow versus time
- Pressure versus time
- Volume versus time.

Loops are the two-dimensional graphic display of two scalar values. There are two loops available for interpretation. They are:
1. Pressure-volume loop **(Fig. 2)**.
2. Flow-volume loop **(Fig. 3)**.

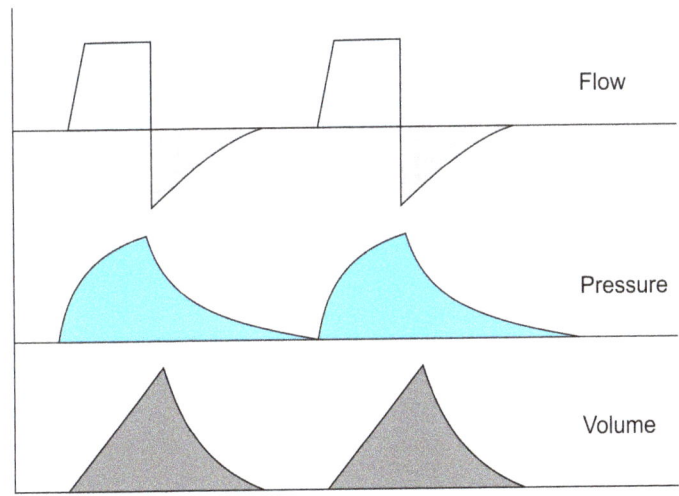

Fig. 1: Scalar graphics.

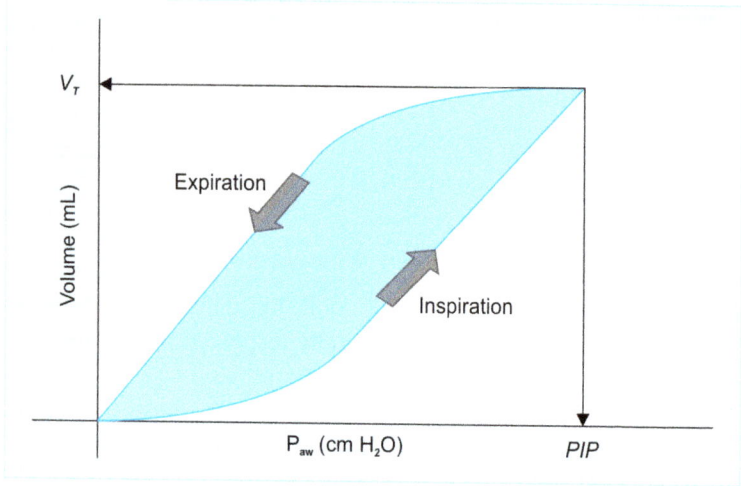

Fig. 2: Pressure-volume loop.
(V_T: tidal volume; PIP: peak inspiratory pressure; P_{aw}: airway pressure)

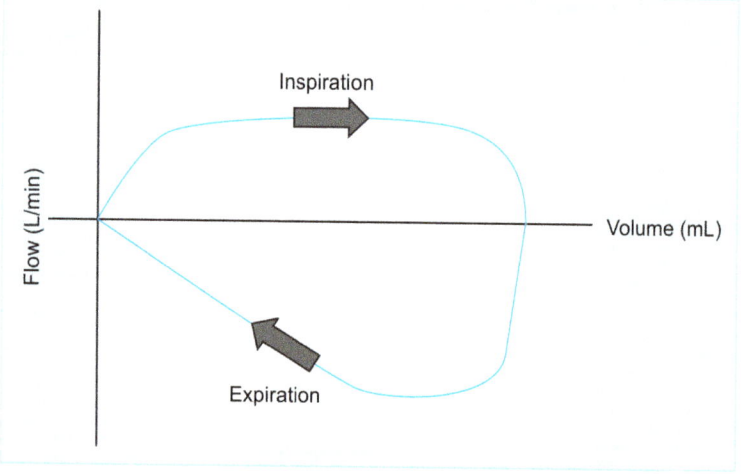

Fig. 3: Flow-volume loop.

SCALAR GRAPHICS

Analysis of scalar graphics is mainly done by the graphical representation with *time* being in X-axis and *flow* in Y-axis.

Basics of *flow* versus *time curve* are shown occurring in the following conditions given here. Individual representations are shown in graphical forms, respectively:

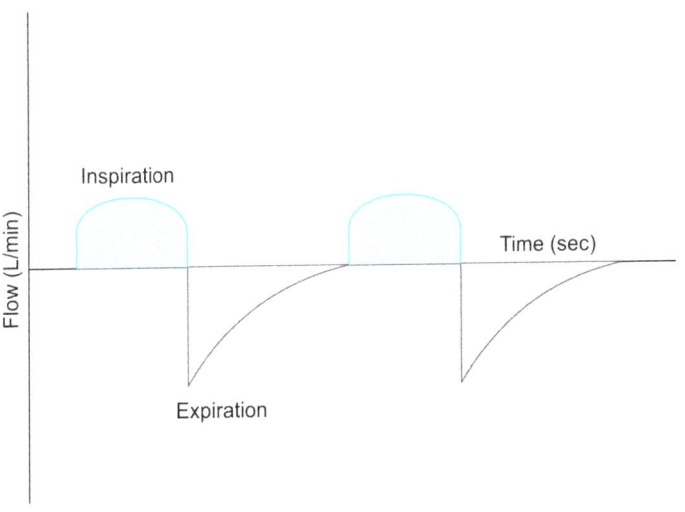

Fig. 4: Spontaneous breath.

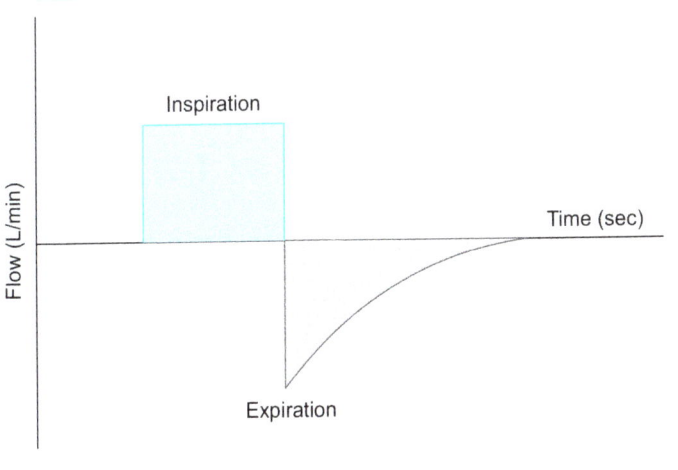

Fig. 5: Mechanical breath.

- Spontaneous breath **(Fig. 4)**
- Mechanical breath **(Fig. 5)**

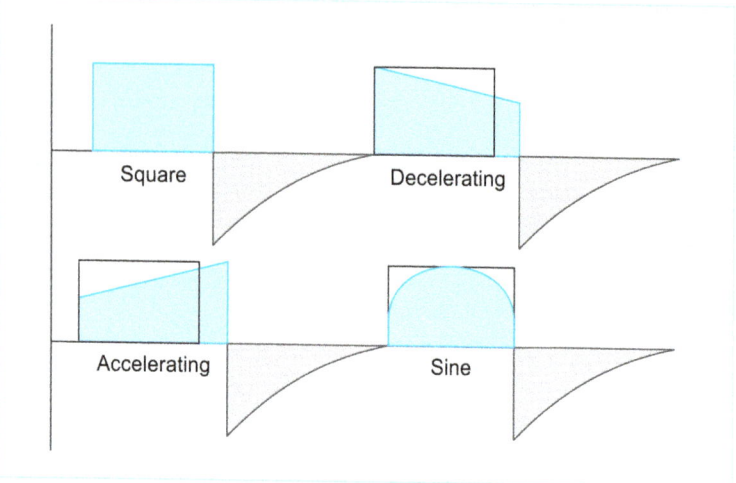

Fig. 6: Flow patterns.

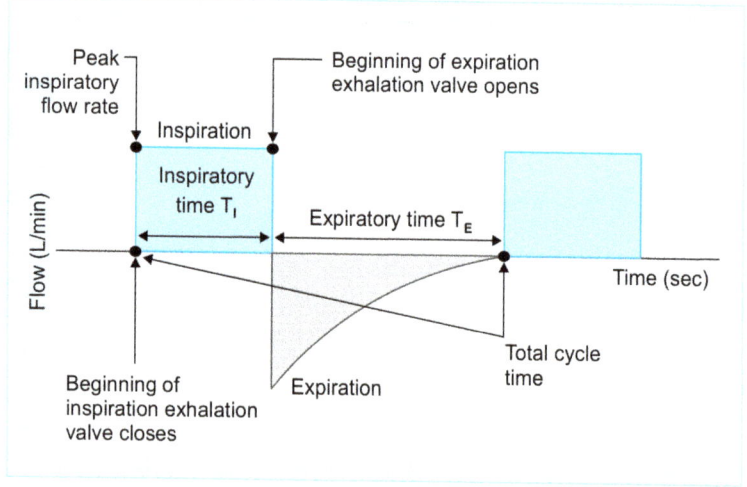

Fig. 7: Inspiratory flow pattern.

- Typical flow patterns **(Fig. 6)**
- Inspiratory flow **(Fig. 7)**
- Expiratory flow **(Fig. 8)**.

Recognition of common abnormalities occurring in ventilated patients can also be interpreted from graphical representations on

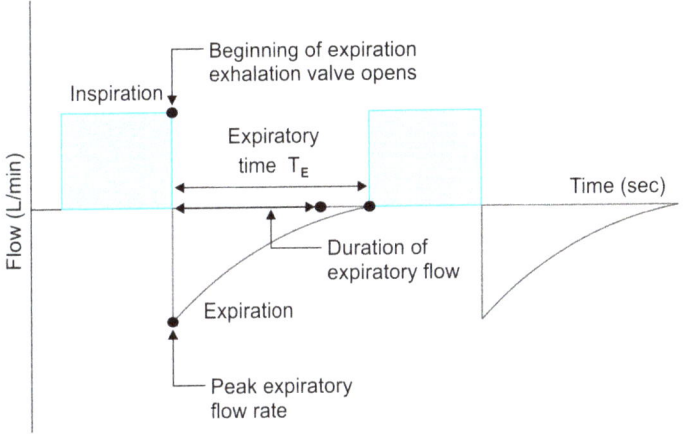

Fig. 8: Expiratory flow pattern.

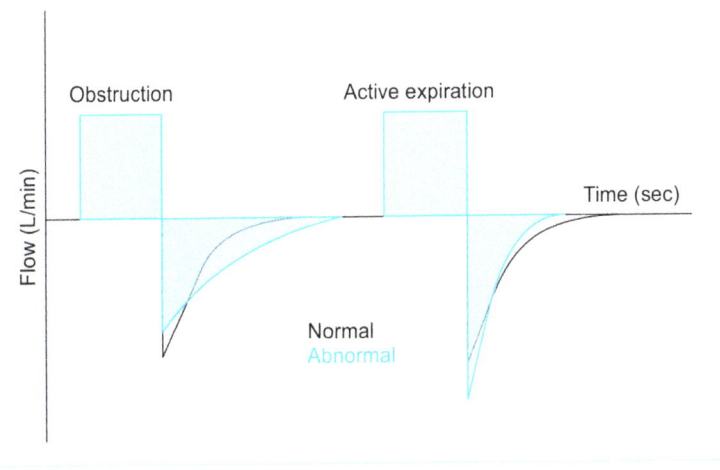

Fig. 9: Obstruction versus active expiration.

the ventilator display in the emergency room. Common problems are as follows:
- Obstruction versus active expiration **(Fig. 9)**
- Response to bronchodilators **(Fig. 10)**
- Air trapping/auto-PEEP (positive end-expiratory pressure) **(Fig. 11)**.

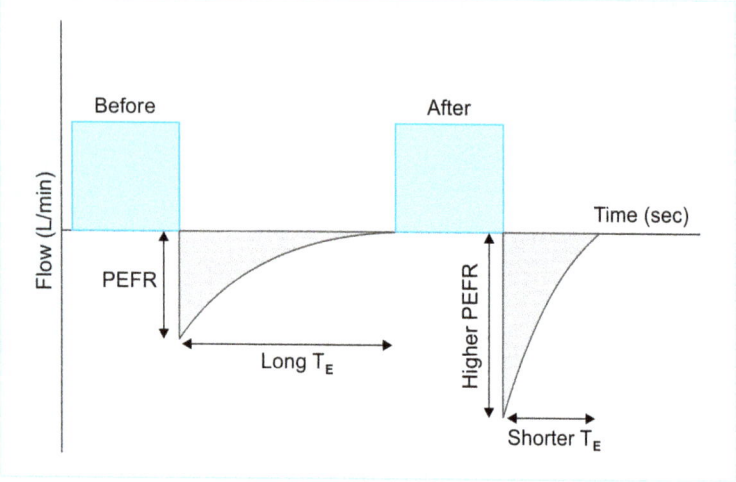

Fig. 10: Response to bronchodilators.
(PEFR: peak expiratory flow rate; T_E: time in expiration)

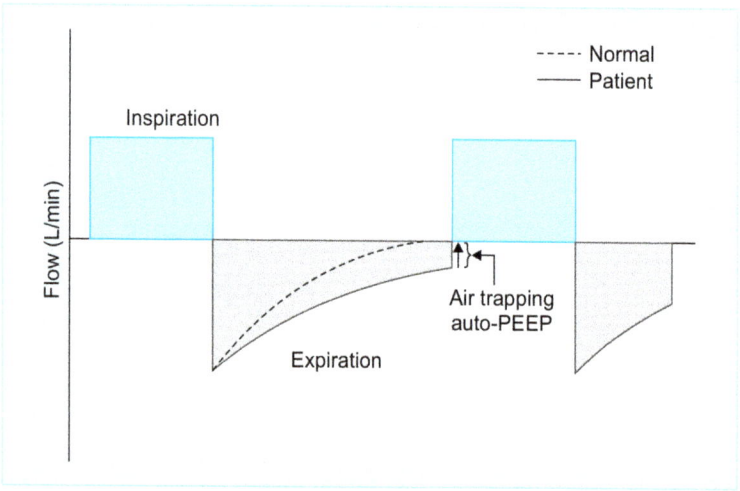

Fig. 11: Air trapping.
(PEEP: positive end-expiratory pressure)

Volume versus Time Curve

Basics of *volume* versus *time curve* are now shown in a graphical form. The graphical representation is done by plotting *volume* in Y-axis and *time* in X-axis. Time taken for inspiration and expiration can be noted in the graph **(Fig. 12)**.

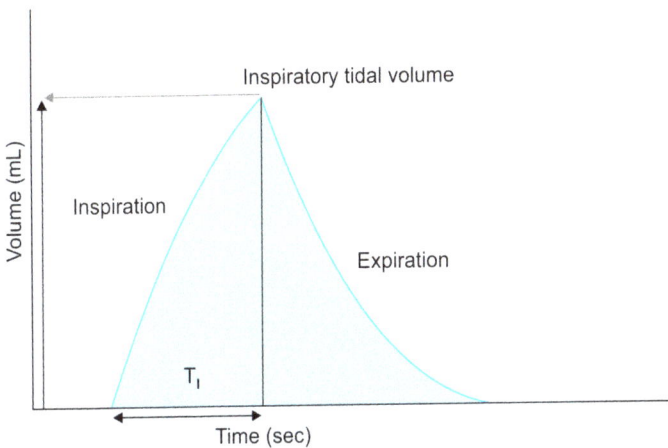

Fig. 12: Volume versus time.
(T_I: inspiratory time)

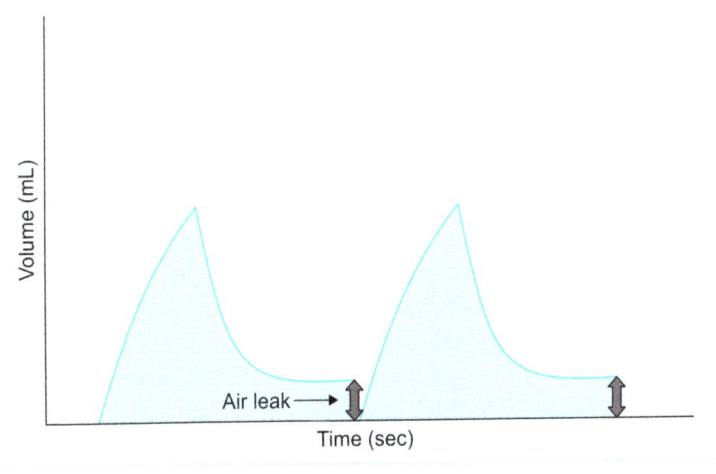

Fig. 13: Air leak.

Recognition of common abnormalities such as: (1) air leak in the ventilating system **(Fig. 13)** and (2) active exhalation **(Fig. 14)** occurring in a ventilated patient can be interpreted by seeing volume versus time relationship graphs.

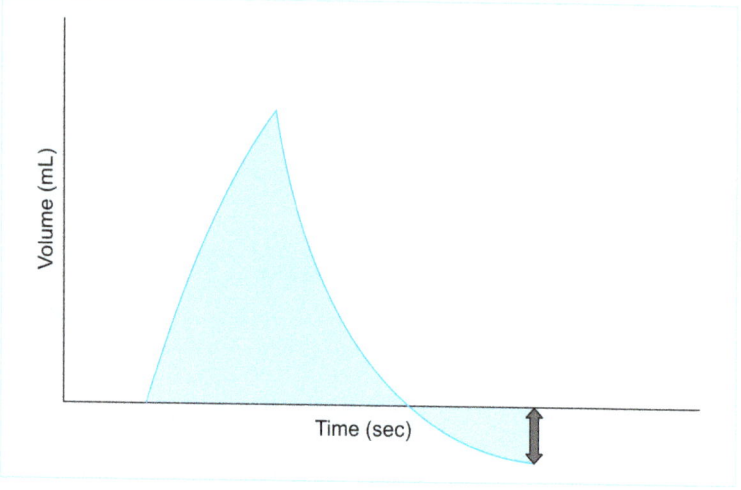

Fig. 14: Active exhalation.

Pressure versus Time Curve

Graphical representation of *pressure* versus *time* curve can also be seen in the ventilator display. Here pressure is plotted in Y-axis and time on X-axis. From these graphical representations, ventilatory parameters can be easily assessed and manipulated as per the need of the patient. Relationship between pressure and time curve in special situations are shown in **Figures 15 to 18**.

Recognition of common problems occurring in a ventilated patient can be done from pressure versus time graphics displayed on the ventilator display. Common abnormalities include: (1) increased airway resistance, (2) effects of high inspiratory flow, (3) decreased lung compliance, and (4) inadequate inspiratory flow.

Pressure versus time graphics demonstrating increased airway resistance and effects of high inspiratory flow are shown in **Figures 19 and 20**.

■ LOOP GRAPHICS

Loop graphics are the two-dimensional graphic display of two scalar values. There are two loops available for interpretation.

Loop graphics can be divided into two groups:
1. Pressure-volume loops.

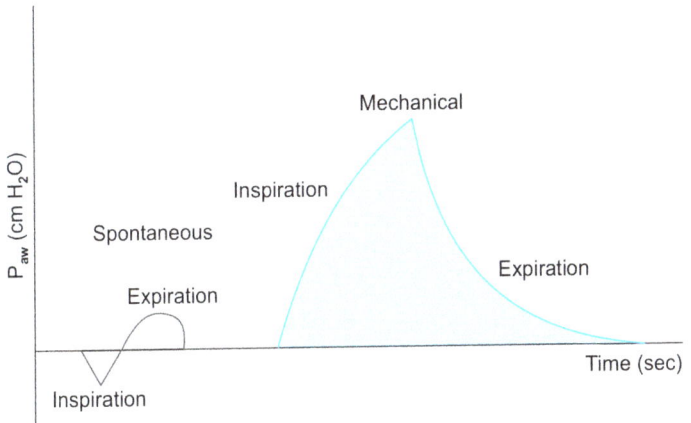

Fig. 15: Spontaneous versus mechanical.
(P_{aw}: airway pressure)

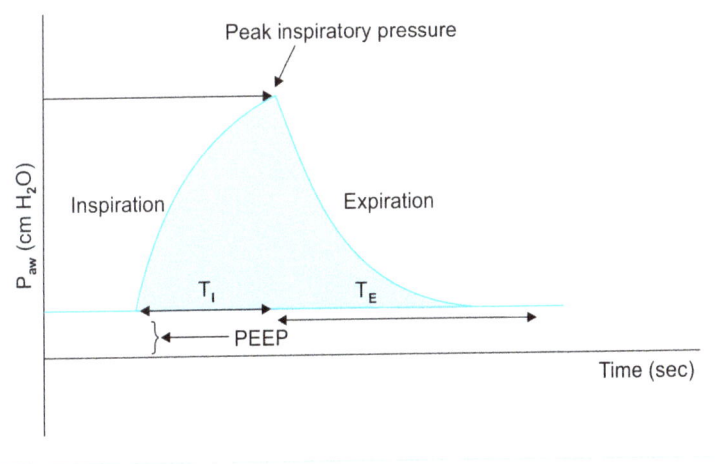

Fig. 16: Mechanical breath.
(P_{aw}: airway pressure; PEEP: positive end-expiratory pressure)

2. Flow-volume loops.

An illustrated view of pressure-volume loops with their basic principles, components, and interpretation of various parameters in relation to physiological and ventilatory parameters are given

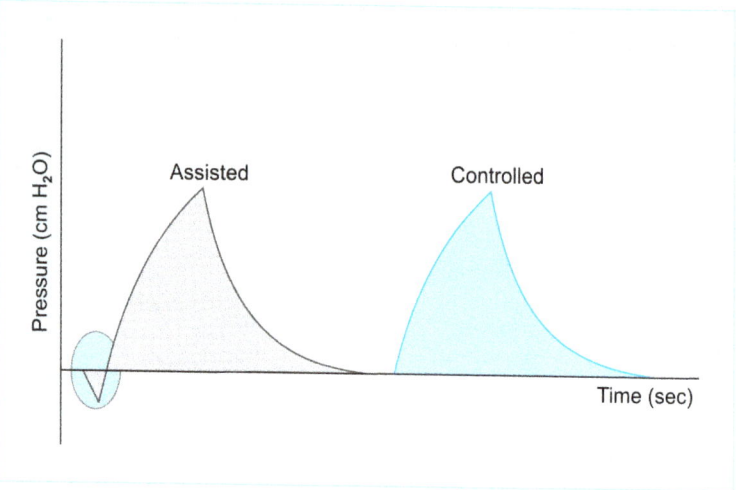

Fig. 17: Assisted versus controlled.

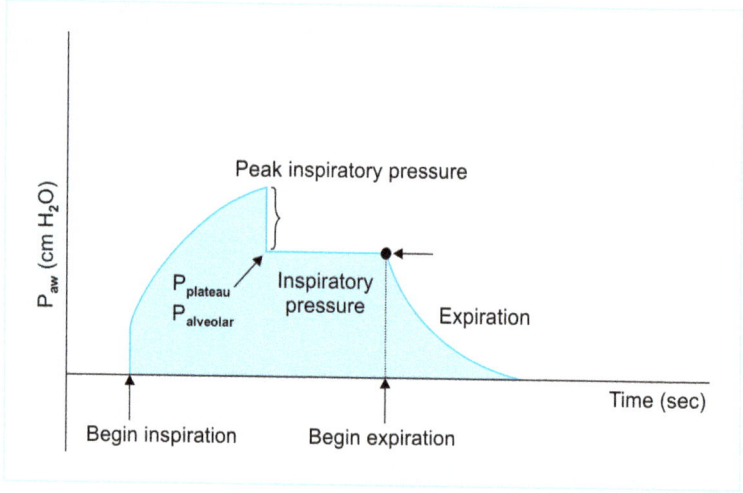

Fig. 18: Components of inflation pressure.
(P_{aw}: airway pressure)

further. Pressure-volume loops explaining (a) Types of breath, (b) Spontaneous-assisted-controlled breaths, (c) Functional residual capacity (FRC) and pressure-volume loops, (d) PEEP and

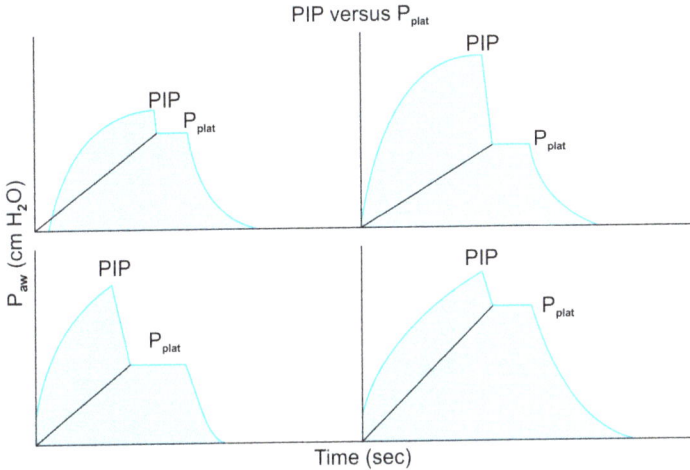

Fig. 19: Increased airway resistance.
(PIP: peak inspiratory pressure; P_{plat}: plateau pressure; P_{aw}: airway pressure)

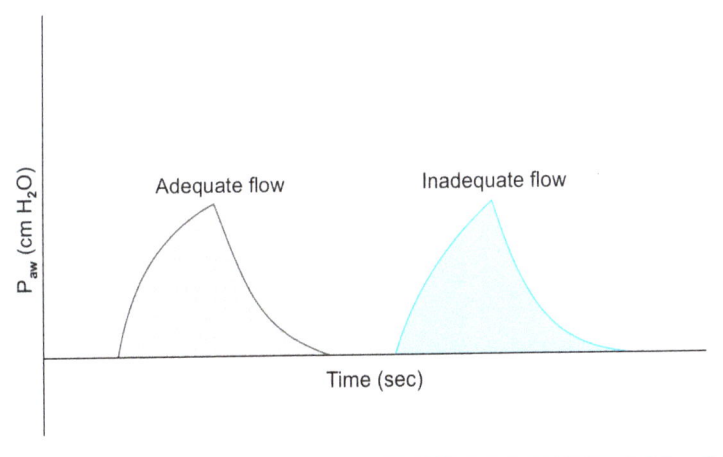

Fig. 20: Inadequate inspiratory flow.
(P_{aw}: airway pressure)

pressure-volume loop, (e) Inflection points, (f) Work of breathing (WOB) are represented systematically in **Figures 21 to 26**.

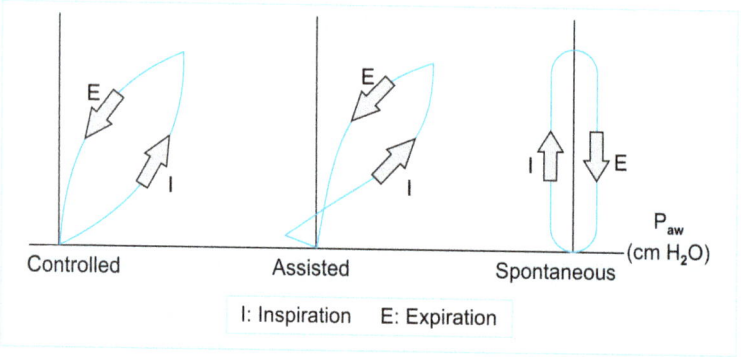

Fig. 21: Types of breath.
(P_{aw}: airway pressure)

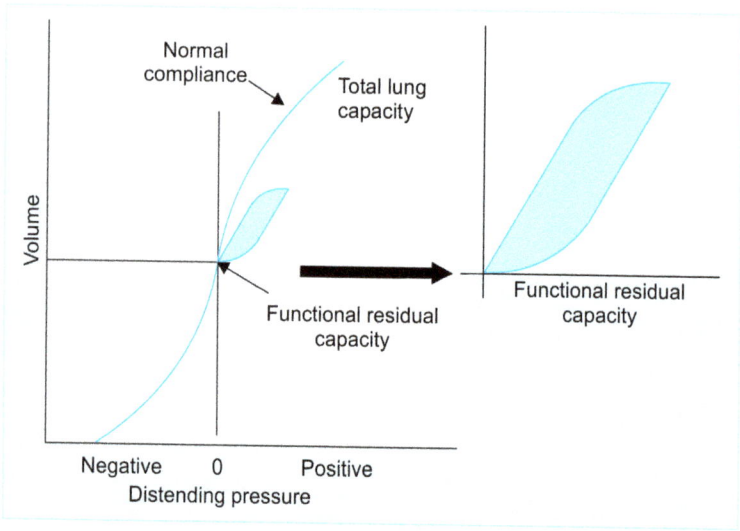

Fig. 22: Functional residual capacity and pressure-volume loop.

The following common abnormalities occurring in course of ventilating a patient can be easily interpreted from pressure-volume loops seen on the display of the ventilator:
- Decreased lung compliance **(Figs. 27A and B)**

CHAPTER 18 | Ventilatory Graphics

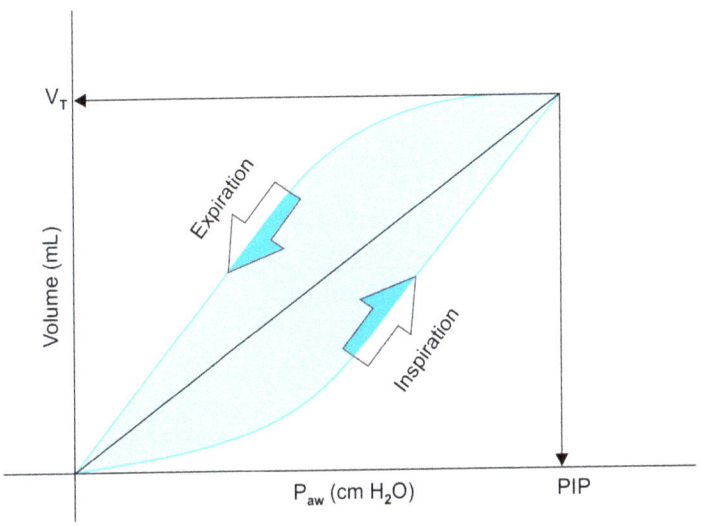

Fig. 23: Components of pressure volume loop.
(PIP: peak inspiratory pressure; P$_{aw}$: airway pressure; V$_T$: tidal volume)

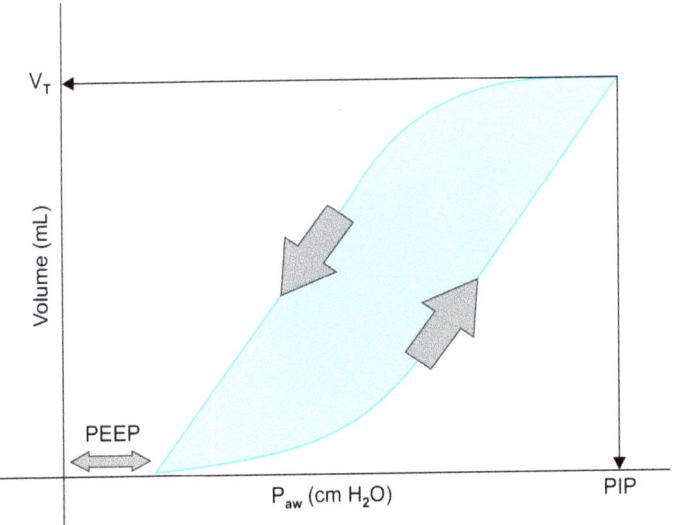

Fig. 24: Positive end-expiratory pressure (PEEP) and pressure-volume loop.
(PIP: peak inspiratory pressure; V$_T$: tidal volume; P$_{aw}$: airway pressure)

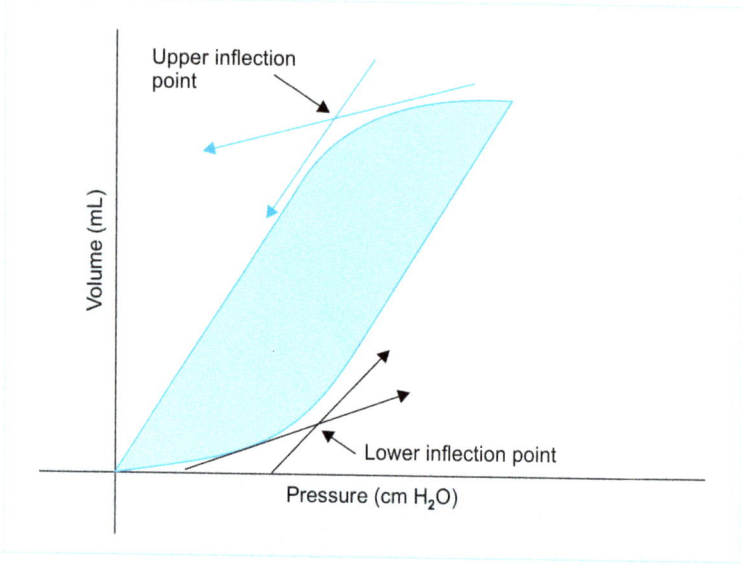

Fig. 25: Inflection points.

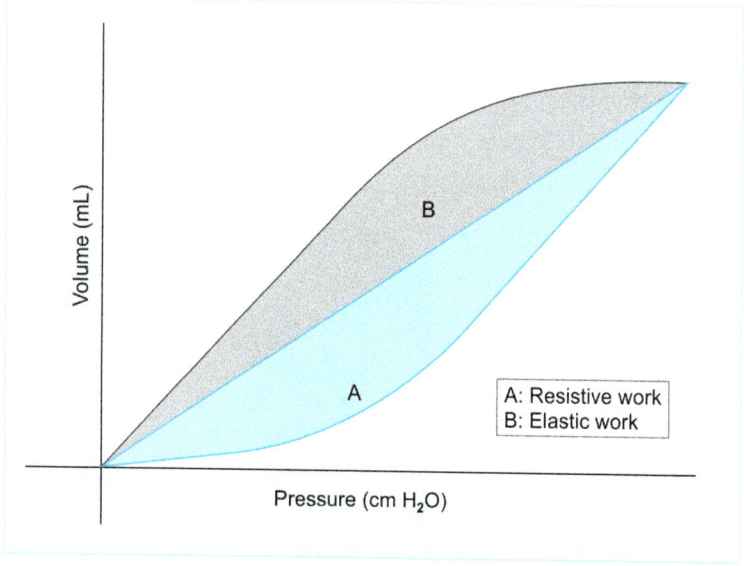

Fig. 26: Work of breathing.

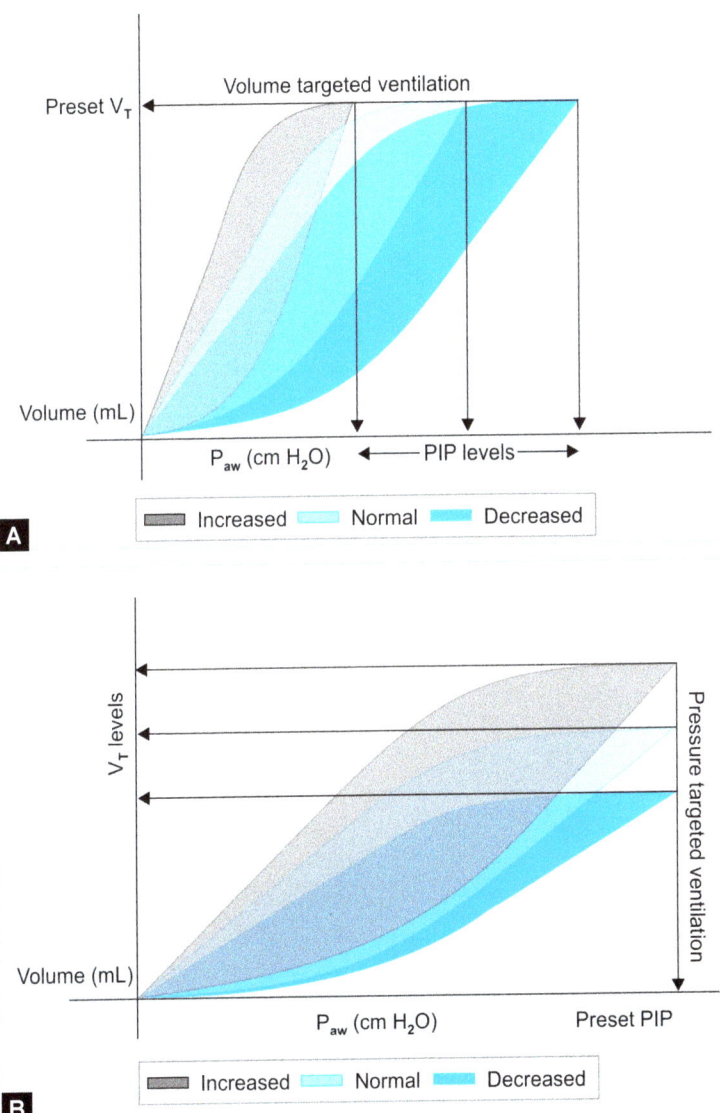

Figs. 27A and B: Lung compliance changes and the pressure-volume loop. (V_T: tidal volume; P_{aw}: airway pressure; PIP: peak inspiratory pressure)

- Increased airway resistance **(Figs. 28 and 29)**
- Alveolar overdistension **(Fig. 30)**

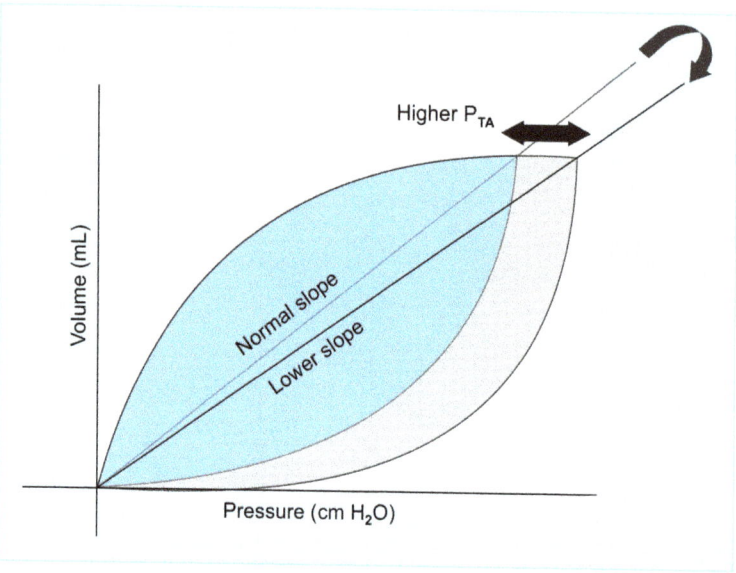

Fig. 28: Increased airway resistance (R_{aw}).
(P_{TA}: transairway pressure)

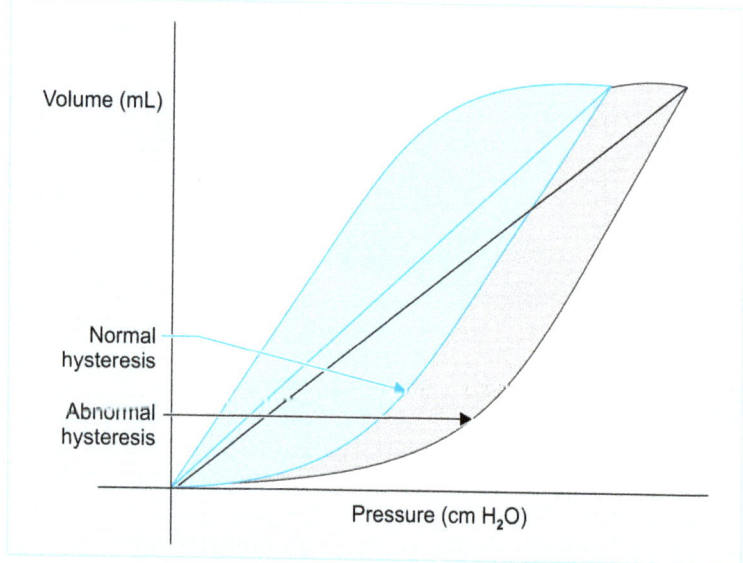

Fig. 29: Hysteresis.

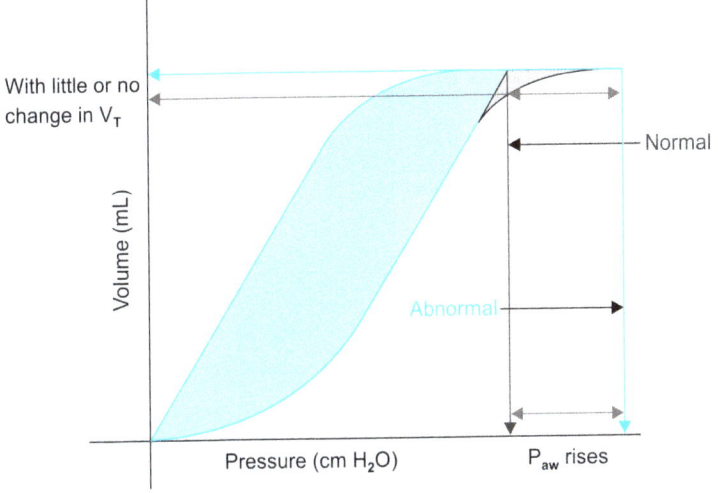

Fig. 30: Overdistension.
(V_T: tidal volume; P_{aw}: airway pressure)

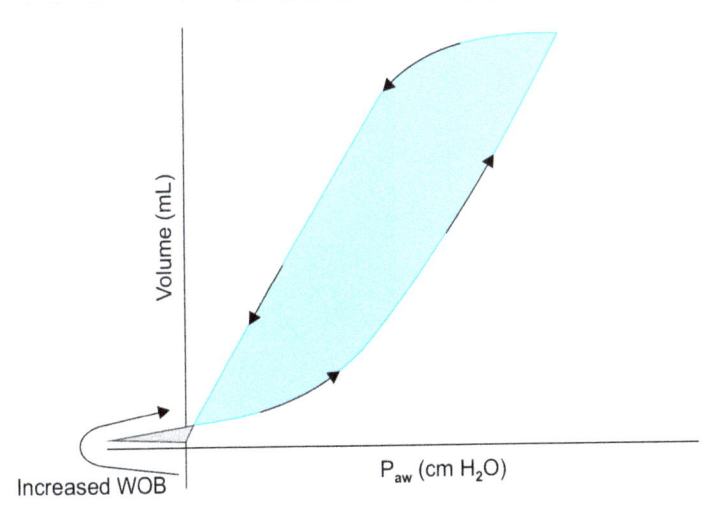

Fig. 31: Inadequate sensitivity.
(WOB: work of breathing; P_{aw}: airway pressure)

- Increased WOB
- Inadequate sensitivity **(Fig. 31)**

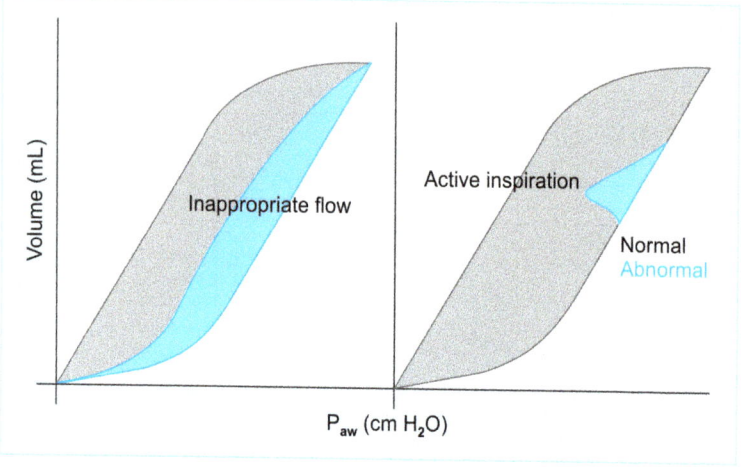

Fig. 32: Inadequate inspiratory flow.
(P_{aw}: airway pressure)

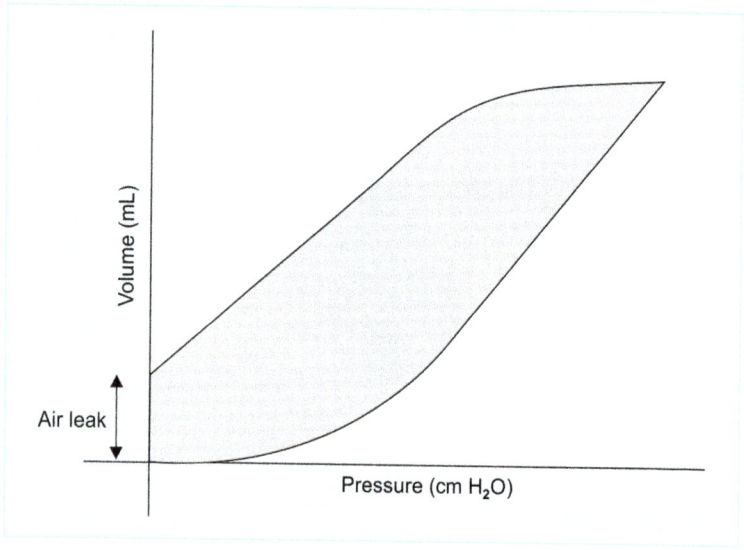

Fig. 33: Air leak in loop.

- Inadequate inspiratory airflow (**Fig. 32**)
- Air leak (**Fig. 33**).

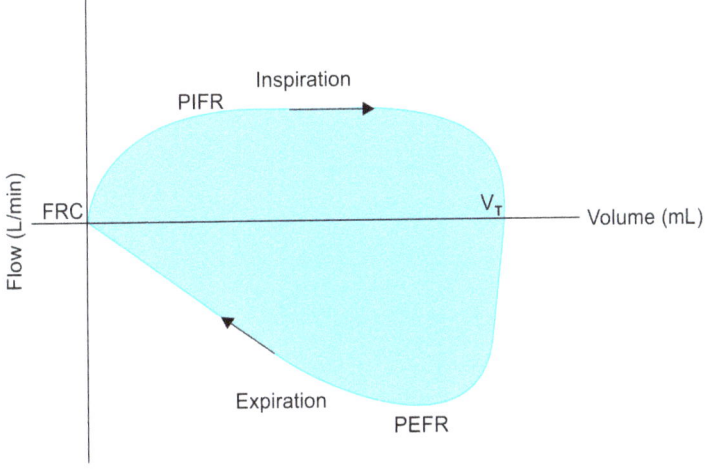

Fig. 34: Flow-volume loop.
(PEFR: peak expiratory flow rate; PIFR: peak inspiratory flow rate; FRC: functional residual capacity; V_T: tidal volume)

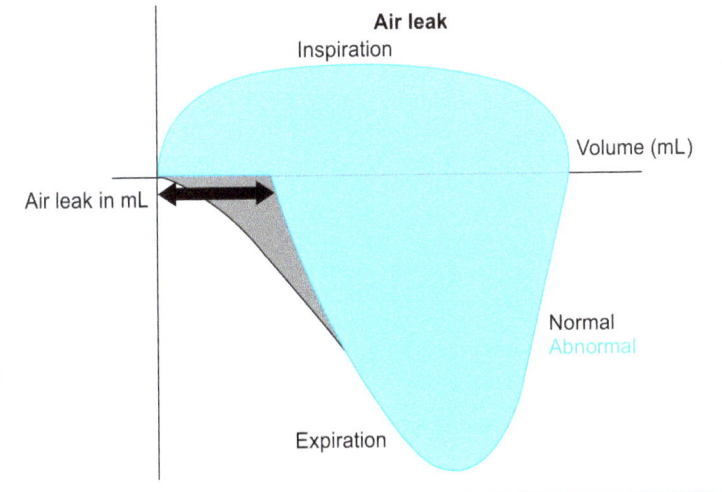

Fig. 35: Air leak in flow-volume loop.

Flow-volume Loop

Flow-volume loop is another type of loop graphics needed for interpretation and management of different patients on ventilators.

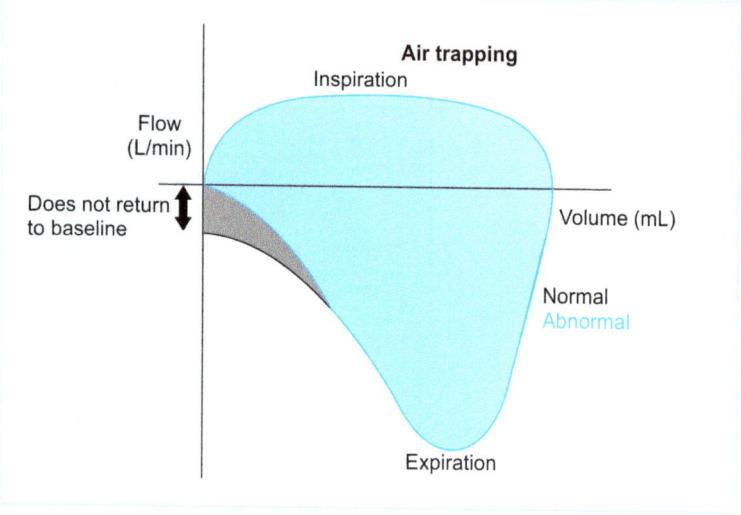

Fig. 36: Air trapping in flow-volume loop.

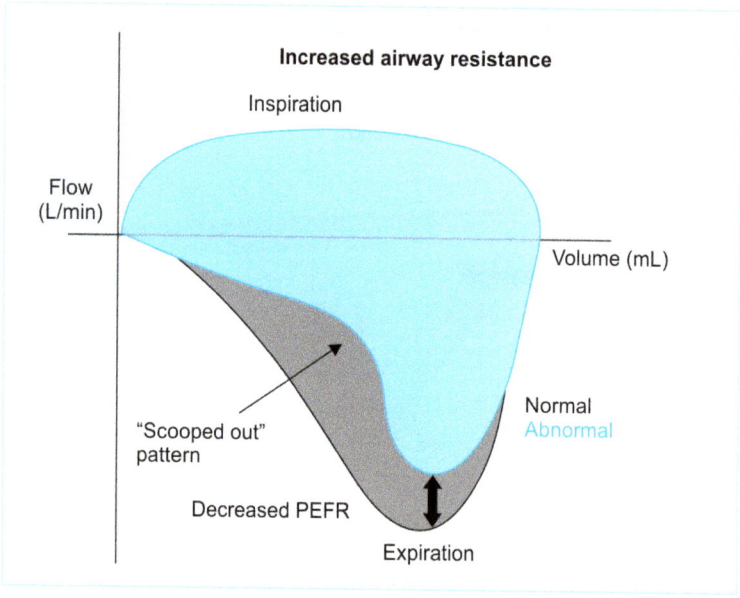

Fig. 37: Increased airway resistance in flow-volume loop.
(PEFR: peak expiratory flow rate)

The components of flow-volume loops are illustrated in **Figures 34 to 38**. Also common problems during ventilation like air leak,

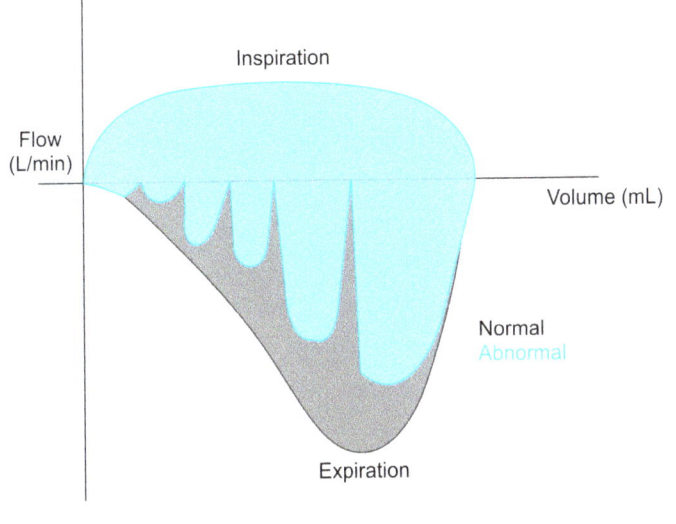

Fig. 38: Airway secretions/water in the circuit.

auto-PEEP, air trapping, increased airway resistance, secretions or condensate accumulating are easily determined with help of this graphics.

Bibliography

1. AARC (American Association for Respiratory Care) clinical practice guidelines. Capnography/capnometry during mechanical ventilation. Respir Care. 1995;40(12):1321-4.
2. Ahmed A, Fenwick L, Angus RM, Peacock AJ. Nasal ventilation vs doxapram in the treatment of type II respiratory failure complicating chronic airflow obstruction Thorax. 1992;47:858.
3. Allardet-Servent J. High-frequency oscillatory ventilation in adult patients with acute respiratory distress syndrome: where do we stand and where should we go? Crit Care Med. 2011;39(12):2761-2.
4. Amato MBP, Barbas CSV, Medeiros DM, Magaldi RB, Schettino GP, Lorenzi-Filho G, et al. Effect of a protective-ventilation strategy on mortality in acute respiratory distress syndrome. N Engl J Med. 1998;338:347-54
5. Amato MBP, Meade MO, Slutsky AS, Brochard L, Costa ELV, Schoenfeld DA, et al. Driving pressure and survival in the acute respiratory distress syndrome. N Engl J Med. 2015;372:747-55.
6. Ambrosino N, Foglio K, Rubini F, Clini E, Nava S, Vitacca M. Non-invasive mechanical ventilation in acute respiratory failure due to chronic obstructive airways disease: correlates for success. Thorax. 1995;50:755-7.
7. Angus RM, Ahmed AA, Fenwick LJ, Peacock AJ. Comparison of the acute effects on gas exchange of nasal ventilation and doxapram in exacerbations of chronic obstructive pulmonary disease. Thorax. 1996;51:1048-50 (published erratum Thorax 1997;52:204).
8. Antonelli M, Conti G, Bufi M, Costa MG, Lappa A, Rocco M, et al. Non-invasive ventilation for treatment of acute respiratory failure in patients undergoing solid organ transplantation: a randomized trial. JAMA. 2000;283:235-41.
9. Antonelli M, Conti G, Rocco M, Bufi M, De Blasi RA, Vivino G, et al. A comparison of noninvasive positive-pressure ventilation and conventional mechanical ventilation in patients with acute respiratory failure. N Engl J Med. 1998;339:429-35.
10. Appendini I, Patessio A, Zanaboni S, Carone M, Gukov B, Donner CF, Rossi A. Physiologic effects of positive end-expiratory pressure and mask pressure support during exacerbations of chronic obstructive pulmonary disease. Am J Respir Crit Care Med. 1994;149:1069-76.
11. Bailey P, Thomsen GE, Spuhler VJ, Blair R, Jewkes J, Bezdjian L, et al. Early activity is feasible and safe in patients of acute respiratory failure. Crit Care Med. 2007;35(1):139-45.

12. Barbe F, Togores B, Rubi M, Pons S, Maimo A, Agusti AG. Noninvasive ventilatory support does not facilitate recovery from acute respiratory failure in chronic obstructive pulmonary disease. Eur Respir J. 1996;9:1240-5.
13. Baum M, Benzer H, Putensen C, Koller W, Putz G. Biphasic positive airway pressure (BIPAP): a new form of augmented ventilation. Der Anesthesist. 1989;38(9):452-8.
14. Bellani G, Laffey JG, Pham T, Fan E, Brochard L, Esteban A, et al. Epidemiology, care, mortality of patients with acute respiratory distress syndrome in intensive care units in 50 countries. JAMA. 2016;315(8):788-800.
15. Benhamou D, Girault C, Faure C, Portier F, Muir JF. Nasal mask ventilation in acute respiratory failure: experience in elderly patients. Chest. 1992;102:912-7.
16. Benzer H. Ventilatory support by intermittent changes in PEEP levels. 4th European Congress on Intensive Care Medicine. Baveno-Stresa. 1988.
17. Bersten AD, Holt AW, Vedig AE, Skowronski GA, Baggoley CJ. Treatment of severe cardiogenic pulmonary edema with continuous positive airway pressure delivered by face mask. N Engl J Med. 1991;325:1825-30.
18. Bhatia SL. The vital capacity of the lungs. Ind Med Gaz. 1929;64(9):519-21.
19. Blanch L, Villagra A, Sales B, Montanya J, Lucangelo U, Luján M, et al. Asynchronies during mechanical ventilation associated with mortality. Intensive Care Med. 2015;41(4):633-41.
20. Bolliger CT, Van Eeden SF. Treatment of multiple rib fractures. Randomized controlled trial comparing ventilatory with nonventilatory management. Chest. 1990;97:943-8.
21. Bonanno PC. Swallowing dysfunction after tracheostomy. Ann Surg. 1971;174(1):29-33.
22. Bott J, Baudouin SV, Moxham J. Nasal intermittent positive pressure ventilation in the treatment of respiratory failure in obstructive sleep apnoea. Thorax. 1991;46:457-8.
23. Bott J, Carroll MP, Conway JH, Keilty SE, Ward EM, Brown AM, et al. Randomised controlled trial of nasal ventilation in acute ventilatory failure due to chronic obstructive airways disease. Lancet. 1993;341:1555-7.
24. Bradley Dosher W, Loomis EC, Richardson SL, Crowell JA, Waltman RD, Miller LD, et al. Effects of multidisciplinary team on ventilator associated pneumonia rates. Crit Care Res Pract. 2014;2014:682621.
25. Brett A, Sinclair DG. Use of continuous positive airway pressure in the management of community acquired pneumonia. Thorax. 1993;48:1280-1.
26. Brochard L, Isabey D, Piquet J, Amaro P, Mancebo J, Messadi AA, et al. Reversal of acute exacerbations of chronic obstructive lung disease by inspiratory assistance with a face mask. N Engl J Med. 1990;323:1523-30.
27. Brochard L, Mancebo J, Wysocki M, Lafaso F, Conti G, Rauss A, et al. Noninvasive ventilation for acute exacerbations of chronic obstructive pulmonary disease. N Engl J Med. 1995;333:817-22.

Bibliography

28. Brower RG, Lanken PN, MacIntyre N, Matthay MA, Morris A, Ancukiewicz M. Higher versus lower positive end-expiratory pressures in patients with the acute respiratory distress syndrome. N Engl J Med. 2004;351(4):327-36.
29. Brown J, Jones D, Mikelsons C, Paul EA, Wedzicha JA. Using nasal intermittent positive pressure ventilation on a general respiratory ward. J R Coll Physicians Lond. 1998;32:219-24.
30. Brown LK, Javaheri S. Positive airway pressure device technology past and present: What's in the "black box"? Sleep Med Clin. 2017;12(4):501-15.
31. Bunburaphomg T, Imanaka H, Nishimura M, Hess D, Kacmarek RM. Performance characteristics of bilevel pressure ventilators: a lung model study. Chest. 1997;111:1050-60.
32. Burja S, Belec T, Bizjak N, Mori J, Markota A, Sinkovič A. Efficacy of a bundle approach in preventing the incidence of ventilator associated pneumonia (VAP). Bosn J Basic Med Sci. 2018;18(1):105-9.
33. Cabrini L, Landoni G, Oriani A, Plumari VP, Nobile L, Greco M, et al. Noninvasive ventilation and survival in acute care settings: a comprehensive systematic review and metaanalysis of randomized controlled trials. Critical Care Med. 2015;43(4):880-8.
34. Calfee CS, Matthay MA. Recent advances in mechanical ventilation. Am J Med. 2005;118(6):584-91.
35. Campbell GD Jr. Blinded invasive diagnostic procedures in ventilator-associated pneumonia. Chest. 2000;117(4 Suppl 2):207S-11S.
36. Carson SS, Cox CE, Holmes GM, Howard A, Carey TS. The changing epidemiology of mechanical ventilation: a population-based study. J Intensive Care Med. 2006;21(3):173-82.
37. Cassidy MR, Rosenkranz P, McCabe K, Rosen JE, McAneny D. I COUGH: Reducing postoperative pulmonary complications with a multidisciplinary patient care program. JAMA Surg. 2013;148(8):740-5.
38. Celikel T, Sungur M, Ceyhan B, Karakurt S. Comparison of noninvasive positive pressure ventilation with standard medical therapy in hypercapnic acute respiratory failure. Chest. 1998;114:1636-42.
39. Charlesworth M, Elliott MW, Holmes JD. Noninvasive positive pressure ventilation for acute respiratory failure in delirious patients: understudied, underreported, or underappreciated? A systematic review and meta-analysis. Lung. 2012;190(6):597-603.
40. Chastre J, Fagon JY, Bornet-Lecso M, Calvat S, Dombret MC, al Khani R, et al. Evaluation of bronchoscopic techniques for the diagnosis of nosocomial pneumonia. Am J Respir Crit Care Med. 1995;152(1):231-40.
41. Chastre J, Fagon JY. Invasive diagnostic testing should be routinely used to manage ventilated patients with suspected pneumonia. Am J Respir Crit Care Med. 1994;150(2):570-4.
42. Chastre J, Fagon JY. Ventilator-associated pneumonia. Am J Respir Crit Care Med. 2002;165(7):867-903.

43. Chastre J, Trouillet JL, Vuagnat A, Joly-Guillou ML, Clavier H, Dombret MC, et al. Nosocomial pneumonia in patients with acute respiratory distress syndrome. Am J Respir Crit Care Med. 1998;157(4 Pt 1):1165-72.
44. Chatburn RL, Volsko TA, Hazy J, Harris LN, Sanders S. Determining the basis for a taxonomy of mechanical ventilation. Respir Care. 2011; 57(4):514-24.
45. Chatburn RL. Classification of ventilator modes: update and proposal for implementation. Respir Care. 2007;52:301-23.
46. Chen CJ, Li CJ, Tzeng YL, Hsu LN. Successful mechanical ventilation weaning experiences at respiratory care centres. J Nurs Res. 2009;17(2):93-101.
47. Chevrolet JC, Jolliet P, Abajo B, Toussi A, Louis M. Nasal positive pressure ventilation in patients with acute respiratory failure. Chest. 1991;100:775- 82.
48. Chiumello D, Coppola S, Froio S, Gregoretti C, Consonni D. Noninvasive ventilation in chest trauma: systemic review and meta-analysis. Intensive Care Med. 2013;39(7):1171-80.
49. Chopra M, Vardhan V, Chopra D. Recent innovations in mechanical ventilator support. J Assoc Chest Phys. 2015; doi: 10.4103/2320-8775.135108.
50. Christopher KL, Neff TA, Bowman JL, Eberle DJ, Irvin CG, Good JT, et al. Demand and continuous flow intermittent mandatory ventilation systems. Chest. 1985;87:625-30.
51. Confalonieri M, Parigi P, Scartabellati A, Aiolfi S, Scorsetti S, Nava S, Gandola L. Noninvasive mechanical ventilation improves the immediate and long-term outcome of COPD patients with acute respiratory failure. Eur Respir J. 1996;9:422-30.
52. Confalonieri M, Potena A, Carbone G, Porta RD, Tolley EA, Umberto Meduri G. Acute respiratory failure in patients with severe community-acquired pneumonia. A prospective randomized evaluation of noninvasive ventilation. Am J Respir Crit Care Med. 1999;160:1585-91.
53. Consensus Conference. Clinical indications for noninvasive positive pressure ventilation in chronic respiratory failure due to restrictive lung disease, COPD, and nocturnal hypoventilation: a consensus conference report. Chest. 1999;116:521-34.
54. Consequences of feeding for orofacial development and breathing. Jornal de Pediatria. 2016.
55. Conway J, Hitchcock R, Godfrey RC, Carroll MP. Nasal intermittent positive pressure ventilation in acute exacerbations of chronic obstructive pulmonary disease: a preliminary study. Respir Med. 1993;87:387-94.
56. Cook DJ, Walter SD, Cook RJ, Griffith LE, Guyatt GH, Leasa D, et al. Incidence of and risk factors for ventilator-associated pneumonia in critically ill patients. Ann Intern Med. 1998;129(6):433-40.
57. Corbellini C, Trevisan CBE, Villafañe JF, da Costa AD, Vieira SGR. Weaning from mechanical ventilation: a cross sectional study of reference values and the discriminative validity of aging. J Phys Ther Sci. 2015;27(6):1945-50.

58. Corona TM, Aumann M. Ventilator waveform interpretation in mechanically ventilated patients. J Vet Emerg Crit Care. 2011;21(5):496-514.
59. Cowan MJ, Shelhamer JH, Levine SJ. Acute respiratory failure in the HIV-seropositive patient. Crit Care Clin. 1997;13:523-52.
60. Cox CA, Wolfson MR, Shaffer TH. Liquid ventilation: a comprehensive overview. Neonatal Netw. 1996;15(3):31-43.
61. Craven DE, Steger KA. Nosocomial pneumonia in mechanically ventilated adult patients: epidemiology and prevention in 1996. Semin Respir Infect. 1996;11(1):32-53.
62. Dallas J, Skrupky L, Abebe N, Boyle WA 3rd, Kollef MH. Ventilator-associated tracheobronchitis in a mixed surgical and medical ICU population. Chest. 2011;139(3):513-8.
63. Daoud EG. Airway pressure release ventilation. Ann Thorac Med. 2007;2(4): 176-9.
64. De Jonghe B, Lacherade JC, Sharshar T, Outin H. Intensive care unit—acquired weakness: risk factors and preventions. Crit Care Med. 2009;37(10 Suppl):S309-15.
65. De Lucas P, Tarancon C, Puente L, Rodriguez C, Tafay E, Monturiol JM. Nasal continuous positive airway pressure in patients with COPD in acute respiratory failure: a study of the immediate effects. Chest. 1993;104:1694-7.
66. Degraeuwe PL, Vos GD, Blanco CE. Perfluorochemical liquid ventilation: from the animal laboratory to the intensive care unit. Int J Artif Organs. 1995;18(10):674-83.
67. Delclaux C, L'Her E, Alberti C, Mancebo J, Abroug F, Conti G, et al. Treatment of acute hypoxemic nonhypercapnic respiratory insufficiency with continuous positive airway pressure delivered by a face mask: a randomized controlled trial. JAMA. 2000;284:2352-60.
68. DeRiso AJ 2nd, Ladowski JS, Dillon TA, Justice JW, Peterson AC. Chlorhexidine gluconate 0.12% oral rinse reduces the incidence of total nosocomial respiratory infection and nonprophylactic systemic antibiotic use in patients undergoing heart surgery. Chest. 1996;109(6):1556-61.
69. Dexter AM, Clark K. Ventilator graphics: scalars, loops, and secondary measures. Respir Care. 2020;65(6):739-59.
70. Dirkes S. Liquid ventilation: new frontiers in the treatment of ARDS. Crit Care Nurse. 1996;16(3):53-8.
71. Doherty MJ, Greenstone MA. Survey of noninvasive ventilation (NIPPV) in patients with acute exacerbation of chronic obstructive pulmonary disease (COPD) in the UK. Thorax. 1998;53:863-6.
72. Donn SM. Neonatal ventilators: how do they differ? J Perinatol. 2009;29 (Suppl 2):S73-8.
73. Donzelli J, Brady S, Wesling M, Theissen M. Secretions, occlusion status, and swallowing in patients with a tracheotomy tube: a descriptive study. Ear, Nose, Throat J. 2006;85(12):831-4.

74. Downs JB, Stock MC. Airway pressure release ventilation: a new concept in ventilatory support. Crit Care Med. 1987;15(5):459-61.
75. Drakulovic MB, Torres A, Bauer TT, Nicolas JM, Nogue S, Ferrer M. Supine body position as a risk factor for nosocomial pneumonia in mechanically ventilated patients: a randomised trial. Lancet. 1999;354(9193):1851-8.
76. Driks MR, Craven DE, Celli BR, Manning M, Burke RA, Garvin GM, et al. Nosocomial pneumonia in intubated patients given sucralfate as compared with antacids or histamine type 2 blockers. The role of gastric colonization. N Engl J Med. 1987;317(22):1376-82.
77. Edenborough FP, Wildman M, Morgan DW. Management of respiratory failure with ventilation via intranasal stents in cystic fibrosis. Thorax. 2000;55:434-6.
78. Elliott MW, Simonds AK. Nocturnal-assisted ventilation using bilevel airway pressure: the effect of expiratory airway pressure. Eur Respir J. 1995;8:436-40.
79. Elliott MW, Steven MH, Phillips GD, Branthwaite MA. Non-invasive mechanical ventilation for acute respiratory failure. BMJ. 1990;300:358-60.
80. Ellis E, Bye P, Brudere JW, Sullivan CE, et al. Treatment of respiratory failure during sleep in patients with neuromuscular disease: positive pressure ventilation through a nose mask. Am Rev Respir Dis. 1987;135:148-52.
81. Elpern EH, Borkgren Okonek M, Bacon M, Gerstung C, Skrzynski M. Effects of the Passy-Muir tracheostomy speaking valve on pulmonary aspiration in adults. Heart Lung. 2000;29(4):287-93.
82. Esan A, Hess DR, Raoof S, George L, Sessler CN. Severe hypoxemic respiratory failure: part 1—ventilation strategies. Chest. 2010;137(5):1203-16.
83. Esteban A, Anzueto A, Alia I, Gordo F, Apezteguia C, Palizas F, et al. How is mechanical ventilation employed in the intensive care unit? An international utilization review. Am J Respir Crit Care Med. 2000;161:1450.
84. Fabregas N, Ewig S, Torres A, El-Ebiary M, Ramirez J, de La Bellacasa JP, et al. Clinical diagnosis of ventilator-associated pneumonia revisited: comparative validation using immediate postmortem lung biopsies. Thorax. 1999;54(10):867-73.
85. Fagon JY, Chastre J, Hance AJ, Montravers P, Novara A, Gibert C. Nosocomial pneumonia in ventilated patients: a cohort study evaluating attributable mortality and hospital stay. Am J Med. 1993;94(3):281-8.
86. Ferguson T, Gilmartin M. CO_2 rebreathing during BiPAP ventilatory assistance. Am J Respir Crit Care Med. 1995;151:1126-35.
87. Frawley PM, Habashi NM. Airway pressure release ventilation: theory and practice. AACN Clin Issues. 2001;12:234-46.
88. Gachot B, Clair B, Wolff M, Regnier B, Vachon F. Continuous positive airway pressure by face mask or mechanical ventilation in patients with human immunodeficiency virus infection and severe Pneumocystis carinii pneumonia. Intensive Care Med. 1992;18:155-9.
89. Gandevia B. The breath of life: an essay on the earliest history of respiration—Part ii. Aust J Physiother. 2014;16(2):57-69.

Bibliography

90. Gaseous Exchange Systems. [online] Available from: http://www.biologymad.com/resources/M6GasExchange.pdf [Last accessed February, 2021].
91. Geiseler J, Kelbel C. Weaning from mechanical ventilation. Weaning categories and weaning concepts. Med Klin Intensivmed Notfmed. 2016;111(3):208-14
92. Georgopoulos D, Roussos C. Control of breathing in mechanically ventilated patients. Eur Respir J. 1996;9(10):2151-60.
93. Germec-Cakan D, Taner T, Akan S. Uvulo-glossopharyngeal dimensions in non-extraction, extraction with minimum anchorage, and extraction with maximum anchorage. Eur J Orthod. 2011;33(5):515-20.
94. Girault C, Richard JC, Chevron V, Tamion F, Pasquis P, Leroy J, et al. Comparative physiologic effects of noninvasive assist-control and pressure support ventilation in acute hypercapnic respiratory failure. Chest. 1997;111:1639-48.
95. Goldberg P, Reissmann H, Maltais F, Ranieri M, Gottfried SB. Efficacy of noninvasive CPAP in COPD with acute respiratory failure. Eur Respir J. 1995;8:1894-900.
96. Gonzalez-Bermejo J, Janssens JP, Rabec C, Perrin C, Lofaso F, Langevin B, et al. Framework for patient–ventilator asynchrony during long-term noninvasive ventilation. Thorax. 2019;74(7). [online] Available from: http://dx.doi.org/10.1136/thoraxjnl-2018-213022 [Last accessed February, 2021].
97. Greenspan JS. Physiology and clinical role of liquid ventilation therapy. J Perinatol. 1996;16(2 Pt 2 Su):S47-52.
98. Gregg RW, Friedman BC, Williams JF, McGrath BJ, Zimmerman JE. Continuous positive airway pressure by face mask in Pneumocystis carinii pneumonia. Crit Care Med. 1990;18:21-4.
99. Grossbach I, Chlan L, Tracy MF. Overview of mechanical ventilator support and management of patient- and ventilator-related responses. Crit Care Nurse. 2011;31(3):30-44.
100. Grübler MR, Wigger O, Berger D, Blöchlinger S. Basic concepts of heart–lung interactions during mechanical ventilation. Swiss Med Wkly. 2017;147:w14491.
101. Guthrie SO, Lynn C, Lafleur BJ, Donn SM, Walsh WF. A crossover analysis of mandatory minute ventilation compared to synchronized intermittent mandatory ventilation in neonates. Journal of Perinatology: Official Journal of the California Perinatal Association. 2005;25(10):643-6.
102. Haworth CS, Dodd ME, Woodcock AA, Woodcock AA, Webb AK. Pneumothorax in adults with cystic fibrosis dependent on nasal intermittent positive pressure ventilation (NIPPV): a management dilemma. Thorax. 2000;55:620-2.
103. Henzler D. What on earth is APRV?. Critical Care (London, England) 2011;15(1):115.

104. Hering R, Zinserling J, Wrigge H, Varelmann D, Berg A, Kreyer S, et al. Effects of spontaneous breathing during airway pressure release ventilation on respiratory work and muscle blood flow in experimental lung injury. Chest. 2005;128(4):29918.
105. Heyland DK, Drover JW, MacDonald S, Novak F, Lam M. Effect of postpyloric feeding on gastroesophageal regurgitation and pulmonary microaspiration: results of a randomized controlled trial. Crit Care Med. 2001;29(8):1495-501.
106. Hilbert G, Gruson D, Vargas F, Valentine R, Gbikpi-Benissan G, Dupon M, et al. Noninvasive ventilation in immunosuppressed patients with pulmonary infiltrates, fever, and acute respiratory failure. N Engl J Med. 2001;344:481-7.
107. Hilbert G, Gruson D, Vargas F, Valentino R, Portel L, Gipki Berisssan G, et al. Noninvasive ventilation for acute respiratory failure: quite low time consumption for nurses. Eur Respir J. 2000;16:710-16.
108. Hodson ME, Madden BP, Steven MH, Trang VT, Yacoub MH. Non-invasive mechanical ventilation for cystic fibrosis patients: a potential bridge to transplantation. Eur Respir J. 1991;4:524-7.
109. Hoffmann B, Welte T. The use of noninvasive pressure support ventilation for severe respiratory insufficiency due to pulmonary oedema. Intensive Care Med. 1999;25:15-20.
110. Hormann C, Baum M, Putensen C, Mutz NJ, Benzer H. Biphasic positive airway pressure (BIPAP): a new mode of ventilatory support. Eur J Anaesthesiol. 1994;11(1):37-42.
111. Hurst JM, DeHaven CB, Branson RD. Use of CPAP mask as the sole mode of ventilatory support in trauma patients with mild-to-moderate respiratory insufficiency. J Trauma. 1985;25:1065-8.
112. Kaplan LJ, Bailey H, Formosa V. Airway pressure release ventilation increases cardiac performance in patients with acute lung injury/adult respiratory distress syndrome. Crit Care. 2001;5(4):221-6.
113. Kashuk JL, Moore EE, Price CS, Zaw-Mon C, Nino T, Haenel J, et al. Patterns of early and late ventilator-associated pneumonia due to methicillin-resistant Staphylococcus aureus in a trauma population. J Trauma. 2010;69(3):519-22.
114. Keenan JC, Marini JJ. Under pressure. Ann Am Thoracic Soc. 2013;10(3). https://doi.org/10.1513/AnnalsATS.201303-049EM.
115. Kerby G, Mayer L, Pingleton SK. Nocturnal positive pressure ventilation via nasal mask. Am Rev Respir Dis. 1987;135:738-40.
116. Kesten S, Rebuck AS. Nasal continuous positive airway pressure in Pneumocystis carinii pneumonia. Lancet. 1988;ii:1414-5.
117. Klompas M, Branson R, Eichenwald EC, Greene LR, Howell MD, Lee G. Strategies to prevent ventilator-associated pneumonia in acute care hospitals: 2014 Update. Infect Control Hosp Epidemiol. 2014;5(8):915-36.

118. Knebel AR, Janson-Bjerklie SL, Malley JD, Wilson AG, Marini JJ. Comparison of breathing comfort during weaning with two ventilator modes. Am J Crit Care. 2015;149(1). https://doi.org/10.1164/ajrccm.149.1.8111572.
119. Kollef MH. Ventilator-associated pneumonia: a multivariate analysis. JAMA. 1993;270(16):1965-70.
120. Kramer N, Meyer TJ, Meharg J, Cace RD, Hill NS. Randomized, prospective trial of noninvasive positive pressure ventilation in acute respiratory failure. Am J Respir Crit Care Med. 1995;151:1799-806.
121. Lacherade JC, De Jonghe B, Guezennec P, Debbat K, Hayon J, Monsel A, et al. Intermittent subglottic secretion drainage and ventilator-associated pneumonia: a multicenter trial. Am J Respir Crit Care Med. 2010;182(7): 910-7.
122. Lapinsky SE, Mount DB, Mackey D, Grossman RF. Management of acute respiratory failure due to pulmonary edema with nasal positive pressure support. Chest. 1994;105:229-31.
123. Leung P, Jubran A, Tobin MJ. Comparison of assisted ventilator modes on triggering, patient comfort and dyspnoea. Am J Respir Crit Care Med. 1997;155:1940-8.
124. Levitt MA. A prospective, randomized trial of BiPAP in severe acute congestive heart failure. J Emerg Med. 2001;21(4):363-9.
125. Lim TK. Treatment of severe exacerbation of chronic obstructive pulmonary disease with mask-applied continuous positive airway pressure. Respirology. 1996;1:189-93.
126. Lin M, Yang YF, Chiang HT, Chang MS, Chiang BN, Cheitlin MD. Reappraisal of continuous positive airway pressure therapy in acute cardiogenic pulmonary edema: short-term results and long-term follow-up. Chest. 1995;107:1379-86.
127. Lofaso F, Brochard L, Hang T, Lorino H, Harf A, Isabey D, et al. Home versus intensive care pressure support devices. Experimental and clinical comparison. Am J Respir Crit Care Med. 1996;153:1591-9.
128. Lumb A. Nunn's Applied Respiratory Physiology, 8th edition. Philadelphia: Elsevier; 2016.
129. Macintyre N. Counterpoint: is pressure assist-control preferred over volume assist-control mode for lung protective ventilation in patients with ARDS? No. Chest. 2011;140(2):2902.
130. Maeda Y, Fujino Y, Uchiyama A, Matsuura N, Mashimo T, Nishimiura M. Effects of peak inspiratory flow on development of ventilator-induced lung injury in rabbits. Anesthesiology. 2004;101:722-8.
131. MAQUET, Modes of ventilation in SERVO-i, invasive and noninvasive, 2008 MAQUET Critical Care AB, Order No 66 14 692.
132. MAQUET, Modes of ventilation in SERVO-s, invasive and noninvasive, 2009 MAQUET Critical Care AB, Order No 66 61 131.
133. Marini JJ. Tidal volume, PEEP, and barotrauma. An open and shut case? Chest. 1996;109:302-4.

134. Markowicz P, Wolff M, Djedaini K, Cohen Y, Chastre J, Delclaux C, et al. Multicenter prospective study of ventilator-associated pneumonia during acute respiratory distress syndrome. Incidence, prognosis, and risk factors. ARDS Study Group. Am J Respir Crit Care Med. 2000;161(6):1942-8.
135. Martin TJ, Hovis JD, Costantino JP, Bierman MI, Donahoe MP, Rogers RM, et al. A randomized, prospective evaluation of noninvasive ventilation for acute respiratory failure. Am J Respir Crit Care Med. 2000;161:807-13.
136. Masip J, Betbese AJ, Paez J, Vecilla F, Canizares R, Padro J, et al. Non-invasive pressure support ventilation versus conventional oxygen therapy in acute cardiogenic pulmonary oedema: a randomized trial. Lancet. 2000;356:2126-32.
137. Maung AA, Kaplan LJ. Airway pressure release ventilation in acute respiratory distress syndrome. Crit Care Clin. 2011;27(3):501-9.
138. McKibben AW, Ravenscraft SA. Pressure-controlled and volume-cycled ventilation. Clin Chest Med J. 1996;17(3):P395-410.
139. Mead J, Takishima T, Leith D. Stress distribution in lungs: a model of pulmonary elasticity. J Appl Physiol. 1970;28(5):596-608.
140. Medical Devices Agency. Medical device and equipment management for hospitals and community-based organizations. MDA DB9801. London: Medical Devices Agency, 1998.
141. Meduri G, Fox R, Abou-Shala N, Leeper KV, Wunderink RG. Noninvasive mechanical ventilation via face mask in patients with acute respiratory failure who refused endotracheal intubation. Crit Care Med. 1994;22:1584-90.
142. Meduri GU, Abou-Shala N, Fox RC, Jones CB, Leeper KV, Wunderink RG, et al. Noninvasive face mask mechanical ventilation in patients with acute hypercapnic respiratory failure. Chest. 1991;100:445-54.
143. Meduri GU, Conoscenti CC, Menashe P, Nair S. Noninvasive face mask ventilation in patients with acute respiratory failure. Chest. 1989;95:865-70.
144. Meduri GU, Cook TR, Turner RE, Cohen M, Leeper KV. Noninvasive positive pressure ventilation in status asthmaticus. Chest. 1996;110:767-74.
145. Meduri GU, Turner RE, Abou-Shala N, Wunderink R, Tolley E. Noninvasive positive pressure ventilation via face mask. First-line intervention in patients with acute hypercapnic and hypoxemic respiratory failure. Chest. 1996;109:179-93.
146. Meecham Jones DJ, Paul EA, Grahame-Clarke C, Wedzicha JA. Nasal ventilation in acute exacerbations of chronic obstructive pulmonary disease: effect of ventilator mode on arterial blood gas tensions. Thorax. 1994;49:1222-4.
147. Mehta S, Jay GD, Woolard RH, Hipona RA, Connolly EM, Cimini DM, et al. Randomized, prospective trial of bilevel versus continuous positive airway pressure in acute pulmonary edema. Crit Care Med. 1997;25:620-8.
148. Melsen WG, Rovers MM, Bonten MJ. Ventilator-associated pneumonia and mortality: a systematic review of observational studies. Crit Care Med. 2009;37(10):2709-18.

149. Meyer T, Hill N. Noninvasive positive pressure ventilation to treat respiratory failure. Ann Intern Med. 1994;120:760-70.
150. Miller RF, Semple SJ. Continuous positive airway pressure ventilation for respiratory failure associated with Pneumocystis carinii pneumonia. Respir Med. 1991;85:133-8.
151. Miro AM, Shivaram U, Hertig I. Continuous positive airway pressure in COPD patients in acute hypercapnic respiratory failure. Chest. 1993;103:266-8.
152. Morrow LE, Kollef MH, Casale TB. Probiotic prophylaxis of ventilator-associated pneumonia: a blinded, randomized controlled trial. Am J Respir Crit Care Med. 2010;182(8):1058-64.
153. Muscedere JG, Mullen JB, Gan K, Slutsky AS. Tidal ventilation at low airway pressure can augment lung injury. Am J Respir Crit Care. 2017;149(5):1327-34.
154. Nava S, Ambrosino N, Bruschi C, Confalonieri, Rampulla C. Physiological effects of flow and pressure triggering during non-invasive mechanical ventilation in patients with chronic obstructive pulmonary disease. Thorax. 1997;52:249-54.
155. Nava S, Ambrosino N, Clini E, Parto M, Orlando G, Vitacca M, et al. Noninvasive mechanical ventilation in the weaning of patients with respiratory failure due to chronic obstructive pulmonary disease: a randomized controlled trial. Ann Intern Med. 1998;128:721-8.
156. Nava S, Evangelisti I, Rampulla C, Compagnoni ML, Fracchi C, Rubini F. Human and financial costs of non-invasive mechanical ventilation in patients affected by COPD and acute respiratory failure. Chest. 1997;111:1631-8.
157. Newberry DL, Noblett KE, Kolhouse L. Noninvasive bilevel positive pressure ventilation in severe acute pulmonary edema. Am J Emerg Med. 1995;13:479-82.
158. Niederman MS, Torres A, Summer W. Invasive diagnostic testing is not needed routinely to manage suspected ventilator-associated pneumonia. Am J Respir Crit Care Med. 1994;150(2):565-9.
159. Non-invasive ventilation as a systematic extubation and weaning technique in acute-on-chronic respiratory failure. Am J Respir Crit Care Med. 1999;160:86-92.
160. Norris MK, Fuhrman BP, Leach CL. Liquid ventilation: It's not science fiction anymore. AACN Clin Issues Crit Care Nurs. 1994;5(3):246-54.
161. O'Gara B, Talmor D. Perioperative lung protective ventilation. BMJ. 2018;362:k3030.
162. Panchabhai TS, Dangayach NS, Krishnan A, Kothari VM, Karnad DR. Oropharyngeal cleansing with 0.2% chlorhexidine for prevention of nosocomial pneumonia in critically ill patients: an open-label randomized trial with 0.01% potassium permanganate as control. Chest. 2009;135(5):1150-6.

163. Pang D, Keenan SP, Cook DJ, Sibbald WJ. The effect of positive pressure airway support on mortality and the need for intubation in cardiogenic pulmonary edema: a systematic review. Chest. 1998;114:1185-92.
164. Parisi M, Gerovasili V, Dimopoulos S, Kampisiouli E, Goga C, Perivolioti E. Use of ventilator bundle and staff education to decrease ventilator-associated pneumonia in intensive care patients. Crit Care Nurse. 2016;36(5):e1-e7.
165. Patrick W, Webster K, Ludwig L, Roberts D, Wiebe P, Youner M. Noninvasive positive-pressure ventilation in acute respiratory distress without prior chronic respiratory failure. Am J Respir Crit Care Med. 1996;153:1005-11.
166. Patwa A, Shah A. Anatomy and physiology of respiratory system relevant to anaesthesia. Ind J Anaesth. 2015;59(9):533-41.
167. Pham T, Brochard LJ, Slutsky AS. Mechanical ventilation: state of the art. Mayo Clin Proc. 2017;2017;92(9):P1382-400.
168. Pierson DJ. Patient–ventilator interaction. Respir Care. 2011;56(2):214-28.
169. Plant PK, Owen JL, Elliott MW. Early use of non-invasive ventilation for acute exacerbations of chronic obstructive pulmonary disease on general respiratory wards: a multicentre randomised controlled trial. Lancet. 2000;355:1931-5.
170. Plant PK, Owen JL, Elliott MW. One year period prevalence study of respiratory acidosis in acute exacerbations of COPD: implications for the provision of non-invasive ventilation and oxygen administration. Thorax. 2000;55:550-4.
171. Polin RA, Sahni R. Newer experience with CPAP. Semin Neonatol. 2002;7(5):379-89.
172. Prabhakaran P, Sasser WC, Kalra Y, Rutledge C, Tofil NM. Ventilator graphics. Minerva Pediatrics J. 2016;68(6):456-69.
173. Prevedoros HP, Lee RP, Marriot D. CPAP, effective respiratory support in patients with AIDS-related Pneumocystis carinii pneumonia. Anaesth Intensive Care. 1991;19:561-6.
174. Prod'hom G, Leuenberger P, Koerfer J, Blum A, Chiolero R, Schaller MD, et al. Nosocomial pneumonia in mechanically ventilated patients receiving antacid, ranitidine, or sucralfate as prophylaxis for stress ulcer. A randomized controlled trial. Ann Intern Med. 1994;120(8):653-62.
175. Protain AP, Firestone KS, McNinch NL, Stein HM. Evaluating peak inspiratory pressures and tidal volumes in premature neonates on NAVA ventilation. Eur J Pediatr. 2021;180(1):167-75.
176. Pugin J, Auckenthaler R, Lew DP, Suter PM. Oropharyngeal decontamination decreases incidence of ventilator-associated pneumonia. A randomized, placebo-controlled, double-blind clinical trial. JAMA. 1991;265(20):2704-10.
177. Pugin J, Auckenthaler R, Mili N, Janssens JP, Lew PD, Suter PM. Diagnosis of ventilator-associated pneumonia by bacteriologic analysis of bronchoscopic and nonbronchoscopic "blind" bronchoalveolar lavage fluid. Am Rev Respir Dis. 1991;143(5 Pt 1):1121-9.

Bibliography

178. Putensen C, Mutz NJ, Putensen-Himmer G, Zinserling J. Spontaneous breathing during ventilatory support improves ventilation-perfusion distributions in patients with acute respiratory distress syndrome. Am J Respir Crit Care Med. 1999;159(4 Pt 1):1241-8.
179. Putensen C, Zech S, Wrigge H, Zinserling J, Stuber F, Von Spiegel T, Mutz N. Long-term effects of spontaneous breathing during ventilatory support in patients with acute lung injury. Am J Respir Crit Care Med. 2001;164(1): 43-9.
180. Rasanen J, Cane RD, Downs JB, Hurst JM, Jousela IT, Kirby RR, et al. Airway pressure release ventilation during acute lung injury: a prospective multicenter trial. Crit Care Med. 1991;19(10):1234-41.
181. Rasanen J, Heikkila J, Downs J, Nikki P, Vaisanen I, Viitanen A. Continuous positive airway pressure by face mask in acute cardiogenic pulmonary edema. Am J Cardiol. 1985;55:296-300.
182. Rello J, Ollendorf DA, Oster G, Vera-Llonch M, Bellm L, Redman R, et al. Epidemiology and outcomes of ventilator-associated pneumonia in a large US database. Chest. 2002;122(6):2115-21.
183. Rennotte MT, Baele P, Aubert G, Rodenstein DO. Nasal continuous positive airway pressure in the perioperative management of patients with obstructive sleep apnea submitted to surgery. Chest. 1995;107:367-74.
184. Respiratory Therapy Zone. [online] Available from: https://www.respiratorytherapyzone.com/drugs-for-mechanical-ventilation/ [Last accessed February, 2021]
185. Rocker G, Mackenzie MG, Williams B, Logan PM. Noninvasive positive pressure ventilation. Successful outcome in patients with acute lung injury/ARDS. Chest. 1999;115:173-7.
186. Rossi A, Polese G, Brandi G, Conti G. Intrinsic positive end-expiratory pressure (PEEPi). Intensive Care Med. 1995;21:522-36.
187. Royal College of Physicians. Oxygen therapy services guidelines. London: Royal College of Physicians, 2000.
188. Rusterholtz T, Kempf J, Berton C, Gayol S, Tournoud C, Zaehringer M, et al. Noninvasive pressure support ventilation (NIPSV) with face mask in patients with acute cardiogenic pulmonary edema (ACPE). Intensive Care Med. 1999;25:21-8.
189. Sanders AE, Akinkugbe AA, Slade GD, Essick GK. Tooth loss and obstructive sleep apnea signs and symptoms in the US population. Sleep Breath. 2016;20(3):1095-102.
190. Sarina K. Positive end-expiratory pressure in acute respiratory distress syndrome. Curr Opin Crit Care. 2016;22:7-13.
191. Sassoon CS, Del Rosario N, Fei R, Rheeman CH, Gruer SE, Mahutte CK, et al. Influence of pressure- and flow-triggered synchronous intermittent mandatory ventilation on inspiratory muscle work. Crit Care Med. 1994;22:1933-41.
192. Sassoon CS, Zhu E, Caiozzo VJ. Assist-control mechanical ventilation attenuates ventilator-induced diaphragmatic dysfunction. Am J Respir Crit Care Med. 2004;170(6):626-32.

193. Schonhofer B, Sonneborn M, Haidl P, Bohrer H, Kohler D, et al. Comparison of two different modes of noninvasive mechanical ventilation in chronic respiratory failure: volume versus pressure controlled devices. Eur Respir J. 1997;10:184-91.
194. Schuster DP, Klain M, Snyder JV. Comparison of high frequency jet ventilation to conventional ventilation during severe acute respiratory failure in humans. Critical Care Medicine. 1982;10(10):625-30.
195. Sharon A, Shpirer I, Kaluski E, Moshkovitz Y, Milovanov O, Polak R, et al. High-dose intravenous isosorbide-dinitrate is safer and better than BiPAP ventilation combined with conventional treatment for severe pulmonary edema. J Am Coll Cardiol. 2000;36:832-7.
196. Shelledy DC, Rau JL, Thomas-Goodfellow L. A comparison of the effects of assist-control, SIMV, and SIMV with pressure support on ventilation, oxygen consumption, and ventilatory equivalent. Heart and Lung: The Journal of Critical Care. 1995;24(1):67-75.
197. Shivaram U, Cash ME, Beal A. Nasal continuous positive airway pressure in decompensated hypercapnic respiratory failure as a complication of sleep apnea. Chest. 1993;104:770-4.
198. Siempos II, Ntaidou TK, Falagas ME. Impact of the administration of probiotics on the incidence of ventilator-associated pneumonia: a meta-analysis of randomized controlled trials. Crit Care Med. 2010;38(3):954-62.
199. Simonds AK, Elliott MW. Outcome of domiciliary nasal intermittent positive pressure ventilation in restrictive and obstructive disorders. Thorax. 1995;50:604-9.
200. Simonds AK. Equipment. In: Simonds AK (Ed) Non-invasive Respiratory Support. London: Chapman and Hall, 1996;16-37.
201. Singer BD, Corbridge TC. Basic invasive mechanical ventilation. South Med J. 2009;102(12):1238-45.
202. Smallwood CD, Walsh BK. Noninvasive monitoring of oxygen and ventilation. Respir Care J. 2017;62(6):751-64.
203. Smith IE, Shneerson JM. A laboratory comparison of four positive pressure ventilators used in the home. Eur Respir J. 1996;9:2410-5.
204. Solsona JF, Díaz Y, Vázquez A, Gracia MP, Zapatero A, Marrugat J. A study of a new test to predict extubation failure. Crit Care J. 2009;13:R56.
205. Soo Hoo GW, Santiago S, Williams AJ. Nasal mechanical ventilation for hypercapnic respiratory failure in chronic obstructive pulmonary disease: determinants of success and failure. Crit Care Med. 1994;22:1253-61.
206. Spieth PM, Carvalho AR, Guldner A, Kasper M, Schubert R, Carvalho NC, et al. Pressure support improves oxygenation and lung protection compared to pressure-controlled ventilation and is further improved by random variation of pressure support. Crit Care Med. 2011;39(4):746-55.
207. Staudinger T, Bojic A, Holzinger U, Meyer B, Rohwer M, Mallner F, et al. Continuous lateral rotation therapy to prevent ventilator-associated pneumonia. Crit Care Med. 2010;38(2):486-90.

Bibliography

208. Stock MC, Downs JB, Frolicher DA. Airway pressure release ventilation. Crit Care Med. 1987;15(5):462-6.
209. Sutherasan Y, Vargas M, Pelosi P. Protective mechanical ventilation in noninjured lungs: review and meta-analysis. Crit Care. 2014;18:211.
210. Sydow M, Burchardi H, Ephraim E, Zielmann S, Crozier TA. Long-term effects of two different ventilatory modes on oxygenation in acute lung injury. Comparison of airway pressure release ventilation and volume-controlled inverse ratio ventilation. Am J Respir Crit Care Med. 1994;149(6): 1550-6.
211. Techniques and devices for monitoring oxygenation. Respir Care. 2003.
212. Tehrani FT. Automatic control of an artificial respirator. Proc IEEE EMBS Conf. 1991;13:1738-9.
213. Tehrani FT. Automatic control of mechanical ventilation. Part 2: The existing techniques and future trends. J Clin Monit Comput. 2008;22(6):417-24.
214. Tehrani FT. Method and apparatus for controlling an artificial respiratory. US patent 4,986,268, issued January 22, 1991.
215. Teixeira P, Pinto M, Alves L, Henriques AF. Rehabilitation nursing care for the person in context of non-invasive ventilation. [online] Available from: https://www.igi-global.com/chapter/rehabilitation-nursing-care-for-the-person-in-the-context-of-non-invasive-ventilation/256337 [Last accessed February, 2021].
216. Teschler H, Stampa J, Ragette R, Konietzko N, Berthon-Jones M. Effect of mouth leak on effectiveness of nasal bilevel ventilatory assistance and sleep architecture. Eur Respir J. 1999;14:1251-7.
217. The Acute Respiratory Distress Syndrome Network. Ventilation with lower tidal volumes as compared with traditional tidal volumes for acute lung injury and the acute respiratory distress syndrome. N Engl J Med. 2000;342:1301-8.
218. Tobin MJ. Pressure controlled ventilation. In: Principles and Practice of Mechanical Ventilation. New York: McGraw-Hill; 1994.
219. Torres A, El-Ebiary M. Bronchoscopic BAL in the diagnosis of ventilator-associated pneumonia. Chest. 2000;117(4 Suppl 2):198S-202S.
220. Torres A, Gatell JM, Aznar E, el-Ebiary M, Puig de la Bellacasa J, Gonzalez J, et al. Re-intubation increases the risk of nosocomial pneumonia in patients needing mechanical ventilation. Am J Respir Crit Care Med. 1995; 152(1):13741.
221. Trevor AJ, Katzung BG, Masters SB. General anesthetics. In: Katzung and Trevor's Pharmacology: Examination and Board Review, 9th edition. New York: McGraw Hill; 2010. Chapter 25.
222. Truwit JD, Marini JJ. Evaluation of thoracic mechanics in the ventilated patients part 1. Primary measurements. J Crit Care. 1988;3(2):133-50.
223. Vitacca M, Clini E, Rubini F, Nava S, Foglio K, Ambrosino S. Non-invasive mechanical ventilation in severe chronic obstructive lung disease and acute respiratory failure: short-and long-term prognosis. Intensive Care Med. 1996;22:94-100.

224. Vitacca M, Rubini F, Foglio K, Scalvini S, Nava S, Ambrosino N, et al. Non-invasive modalities of positive pressure ventilation improve the outcome of acute exacerbations in COLD patients. Intensive Care Med.1993;19: 450-5.
225. Wagner PD. The physiological basis of pulmonary gas exchange: implications for clinical interpretation of arterial blood gases. Eur Respir J. 2015;45:227-43.
226. Weingart SD. Managing initial mechanical ventilation in the emergency department. Ann Emerg Med. 2016;68:614-7.
227. Weinstein RA. Epidemiology and control of nosocomial infections in adult intensive care units. Am J Med. 1991;91(3B):179S-84S.
228. West JB. A century of pulmonary gas exchange. Am J Respir Crit Care Med. 2014;169(8). [online] Available from: https://doi.org/10.1164/rccm.200312-1781OE [Last accessed February, 2021]
229. Williams LM, Sharma S. Ventilator Safety. Stat Pearls [Internet]. Treasure Island (FL): StatPearls Publishing; 2021.
230. Wood KA, Lewis L, Von Harz B, Kollet MH. The use of non-invasive positive pressure ventilation in the emergency department. Chest. 1998;113:1339-46.
231. Wrigge H, Zinserling J, Hering R, Schwalfenberg N, Stuber F, von Spiegel T, et al. Cardiorespiratory effects of automatic tube compensation during airway pressure release ventilation in patients with acute lung injury. Anesthesiology. 2001;95(2):382-9.
232. Wrigge H, Zinserling J, Neumann P, Defosse J, Magnusson A, Putensen C, et al. Spontaneous breathing improves lung aeration in oleic acid-induced lung injury. Anesthesiology. 2003;99(2):376-84.
233. Wysocki M, Tric L, Wolff MA, Millet H, Herman B. Noninvasive pressure support ventilation in patients with acute respiratory failure. A randomized comparison with conventional therapy. Chest. 1995;107:761-8.
234. Wysocki M, Tric L, Wolff MA, Millet H, Herman B. Noninvasive pressure support ventilation in patients with acute respiratory failure. Chest. 1993;103:907-13.
235. Xu XP, Zhang XC, Hu SL, Xu JY, Xie JF, Liu SQ, et al. Noninvasive ventilation in acute hypoxemic nonhypercapnic respiratory failure: a systematic review and meta-analysis. Crit Care Med. 2017;45(7):e727-33.
236. Yamaguchi K, Tsuji T, Aoshiba K, Nakamura H, Abe S. Anatomical backgrounds on gas exchange parameters in the lung. World J Respirol. 2019;9(2):8-29.
237. Younes M. Proportional assist ventilation, a new approach to ventilatory support. Theory. Am Rev Respir Dis. 1992;145(1):114-20.
238. Zilberberg MD, Shorr AF. Prolonged acute mechanical ventilation and hospital bed utilization in 2020 in the United States: implications for budgets, plant and personnel planning. BMC Health Services Res. 2020;8:242.

Index

Page numbers followed by *f* refer to figure, *fc* refer to flowchart, and *t* refer to table.

A

Academia
  presence of 32
  severe 93
Acid-base balance 76
Acinetobacter 82
Acute respiratory
  distress syndrome 47, 82, 91
  failure 49
Air breathed, volume of 21*f*
Air leak 101*f*, 112
  in flow-volume loop 113*f*
  in loop 112*f*
Air trapping 100*f*
  in flow-volume loop 114*f*
Airway
  epithelium 7
  obstruction stiff lung, normal compliance 26*f*
  pressure 61, 64, 65, 65*f*, 66, 103, 105-107, 111
    release ventilation 47, 48*f*
  protection of 89
  secretions 115*f*
  smooth muscles of 7
Alveolar capillary interface 10, 12*f*
  gas exchange in 13*f*
Alveolar dead space 16
Alveolar interstitium 7
Alveolar overdistension 109
Alveolar-arterial oxygen gradient 14
Amyotrophic lateral sclerosis 90
Anatomical dead space 13
Apnea alarm 78
Apneustic centers 4
Arrhythmias 80, 93
Arterial blood gases 76
Assist control mode ventilation 40, 41*f*
Assisted versus controlled 104*f*
Asthma 88
Asynchrony 42
Atracurium besylate 35
Auto-positive end-expiratory pressure 68, 69, 69*f*
Awake intubations 89

B

Barotrauma 58, 81, 91
Blood, oxygenation of 70
Breath
  clashing of 43, 69
  number of 63
  stacking 43, 69
  types of 106*f*
  volume 62
Breathing
  act of 3
  active 3
  control of 4
  high work of 31
  normal 69
  reduction of work of 38
  work of 108*f*, 111
Bronchoalveolar lavage 83, 84
Bronchodilators, response to 100*f*
Bronchospasm 80

C

Capillary endothelium 11
Capnography 76, 77f
Cardiac arrhythmias 93
Cardiovascular parameters 86
Central chemoreceptors 6
Cerebral cortex 5
Cerebrovascular accident 93
Chronic obstructive
    lung disease 88
    pulmonary disease 49
Cisatracurium 35
Clinical pulmonary infection score 82
    modified 82t
Continuous positive airway pressure 45, 46f, 49, 55, 89
Control mode ventilation 39
Coronary artery disease 93
C-reactive protein 84

D

Decelerating waveform 58, 59f
Diaphragm 7
    descent of 3
Dynamic hyperinflation 88

E

Endotracheal tube 79, 83, 87
    cuff leak 79
    migration 79
    obstruction 79
Enterobacter 82
Epilepsy 93
Espiratory muscle dysfunction 31
Etomidate 37
Exhalation, active 102f
Exhaled air 29
Expiration, active 99f
Expiratory flow 98
    pattern 99f
External intercostal muscle 7

F

Fentanyl 35
Flail chest 89
Flow patterns 98f
Flow profiles 58
Flow-volume loop 113, 113f
    increased airway resistance in 114f
Forced expiratory volume 21
Forced vital capacity 21
Functional residual capacity 106f, 113

G

Gas
    diffusion 11
    solubility 12
Gastric distention 86
General anesthetics, types of 34fc
Guillain-Barré syndrome 90

H

Head injury 89
Heart failures 90
High pressure alarms 77
Humidifiers 30
Hybrid ventilators 51
Hypercapnia 71
Hyperventilation 89
Hypocapnia 90
Hypoventilation 31
Hypovolemic shock 90
Hypoxemia 91
Hypoxia 16, 31
Hysteresis 110f

I

Ideal sedation agent 33
Inadequate inspiratory flow 105f, 112, 112f
Inadequate sensitivity 111f
Increased airway resistance 105f, 109, 110f

Induction agents 36
Inflation pressure, components of 104*f*
Inflection points 108*f*
Inhalational anesthetics 34
Inspiration and expiration
    neuronal control of 8
    time ratio 72
Inspiratory alveolar pressure 48
Inspiratory and expiratory centers 5
Inspiratory breath 73
    duration of 59*f*
Inspiratory flow 98
    pattern 98*f*
    rate 59*f*
        high 88
Inspiratory plateau pressures 76
Inspiratory pressures and flow profiles 57
Inspiratory time 61, 64, 65*f*, 74
Inspired oxygen, fraction of 72
Interface attachments, types of 50*f*
Intermittent mandatory ventilation 42, 42*f*
Intrapleural pressure 3
Intrapulmonary pressure 3
Intrapulmonary shunting 16
Intubation, rapid sequence 35

J

J receptors 7

K

Ketamine 36
Klebsiella 82

L

Loop graphics 102
Lorazepam 35
Low pressure alarm 77, 80
Lower respiratory tract infection 84
Lung 12
    compliance 109*f*
    constants of 25

dead spaces of 13
diffusion distance in 13, 14*f*
injury, ventilator-induced 81
lower part of 67
normal 67
plus chest wall 24
restrictive disease of 21, 22*f*
surface area of 12
upper parts of 67
volumes 19
zones of 18*f*

M

Masks 50
Mechanical breath 97, 97*f*, 103*f*
Mechanical ventilation 27
    drugs for 35, 35*t*
    drugs used during 33, 35
    goals of 91
    initiation of 31
Mechanical ventilator 29
    support 31
Mechanoreceptors 7
Medullary respiratory centers 4
Metabolic alkalosis 86
Methicillin-sensitive *Staphylococcus aureus* 84
Midazolam 35, 36
Minute ventilation 72
Morphine 35
Multidrug resistant 84
Muscles
    abdominal 7
    accessory 8
Myasthenia gravis 90
Myocardial infarction 90

N

Nebulizers 89
Neuromuscular diseases 90
Noninvasive positive-pressure ventilation 49, 50
    complications of 55
    contraindications for 53

selection criteria for 52
weaning from 55
Noninvasive ventilation 49
    failure of 31
Nucleus
    gigantocellularis 8
    parabrachialis medialis 8

O

Obstructive lung diseases 21
Obstructive sleep apnea 49
Open lung concept 47
Oscillatory ventilation, high frequency 47
Overdistension 111f

P

Pancuronium 35
Paralytic agents 37, 86
Parasternal muscles, contraction of 3
Passive breathing 3
Peak expiratory flow rate 100, 113, 114
Peak inspiratory pressure 57f, 105, 107
Perfusion imbalance 13
Peripheral chemoreceptors 6
Permissive hypercapnia 93
Physiological dead space 14
Plateau inspiratory pressure 57, 58
Plateau pressure 88, 105
Pneumocytes, type II 11
Pneumomediastinum 58, 81
Pneumonia 16
Pneumotaxis centers 4
Pneumothorax 58, 81
Poiseuille's law 22
Poliomyelitis 90
Polyvinyl corrugated tubes 29
    interconnecting 30
Pontine respiratory
    centers 4
    group 4
Positive airway pressure
    bilevel 46, 56, 89
    biphasic 65f

Positive end-expiratory pressure 46f, 61, 64, 65f, 66, 67, 67f, 69, 72, 74f, 75, 83, 88, 100, 103, 107f
Pressure
    control mode 75f
    normal 24f
    volume loop, components of 107f
Pressure support 65f, 66, 74f, 75
    ventilation 44, 44f, 52
        criteria for 45
Pressure-controlled 65f
    airway pressure release ventilation 65f
    assist control ventilation 64f, 74
    pressure support ventilation 63, 66f
    ventilation 61, 61f, 62
Pressure-volume loop 96f, 106f, 107f
Propofol 36
Protected specimen brush 83
Pseudomonas 82
Pulmonary arterial hypertension 93
Pulmonary dynamics 21
Pulmonary embolism 16
Pulmonary gas exchange 10
Pulmonary infection 81
Pulmonary mechanics criteria 31
Pulmonary receptors 7
Pulmonary stretch receptors 7

R

Red blood cell 13
Respiration, muscles of 8f
Respirator rate 74f, 75
Respiratory bronchiole 11f
Respiratory centers 4, 5f, 6f
Respiratory cycle 38f, 49, 68
    time 72
Respiratory effectors 7
Respiratory failure, chronic 49
Respiratory muscles 7, 90
Respiratory physiology 19
    compliance 23
    dynamic compliance 25
    static compliance 24

Index

Respiratory rate 61, 64, 65*f*, 71, 86
Respiratory sensors 6
Respiratory system 61
    static volumes of 19*f*
Right bronchus intubation 79
Rocuronium 35, 37

S

Scalar graphics 95*f*
    analysis of 96
Scalene muscles 7
    contraction of 3
Self-extubation 80
Sine waveform 59
Sinusoidal waveform 60*f*
Spontaneous breathing 52, 97, 97*f*
    trial 87
Square waveform 58
Staphylococcus 82
Sternocleidomastoid 7
Succinylcholine 35, 37
Suxamethonium 37
Switch neurons 8
Synchronized intermittent mandatory ventilation 43, 43*f*, 78

T

Tachycardia 86
Thiopentone 36
Thoracic cavity 73
Tidal volume 71, 74, 107
Tooth trauma 80
Total lung volume 20*f*
Tracheoinnominate artery fistula 80
Tracheostomy
    complications 80
    tube 87
Transairway pressure 110
Trigger sensitivity 73

V

Vecuronium 35, 37
Ventilated patients, monitoring of 76

Ventilation
    continuum of 15*f*
    dead spaces of 13
    inverse ratio 73, 92
    prone 92
    proportional assist 52
    rescue modes of 47
Ventilation-perfusion mismatch 15
Ventilator
    alarms 77
    circuit 30*f*
    general settings in 71
    infection-related 83
    management of 84*fc*
    modes of 52
    settings of 74, 75
    type of 51
Ventilator-associated
    complication 83
    events 83*t*
Ventilator-associated pneumonia 81, 83
    prevention of 85, 85*t*
    scoring systems for 82
Ventilator-driven breath 61
Ventilatory complications 79
    in emergency room 79
Ventilatory graphics 95
Ventilatory modes 38
    classification 39
Ventilatory pressure, high 90
Ventilatory strategies 88
    normal 89
Ventilatory support 76
Volume control
    mode 39, 74
    ventilation, basis of 39
Volume guarantee 63
Volutrauma 58, 81, 91

W

Water traps 30
Weaning
    parameters 86
    prerequisites for 87

EU GSPR Authorised Reprsentative
Logos Europe, 9 rue Nicolas Poussin
1700, La Rochelle, France
Phone: +33 (0) 6 67 93 73 78
E-mail: contact@logoseurope.eu

www.ingramcontent.com/pod-product-compliance
Ingram Content Group UK Ltd.
Pitfield, Milton Keynes, MK11 3LW, UK
UKHW021827140426
5217IPUK00016B/1245